Aortic Aneurysm and Aortic Dissection

Edited by Jeffrey Shuhaiber

Published in London, United Kingdom

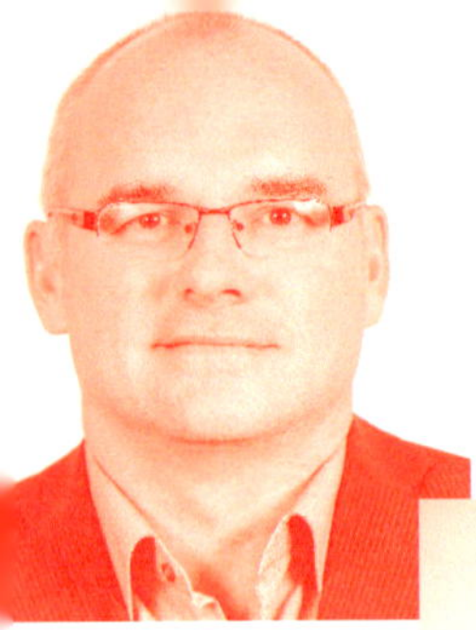
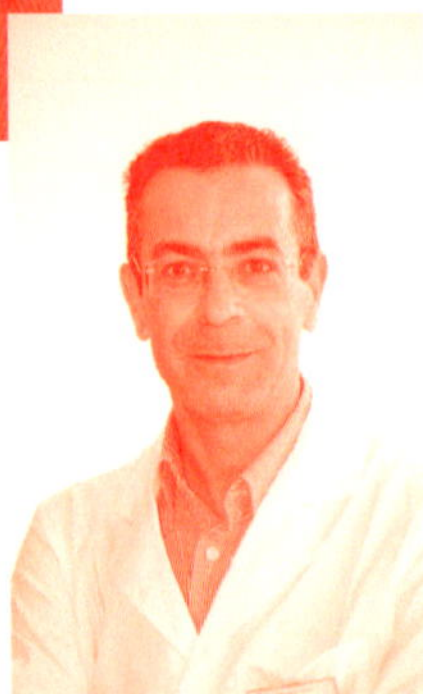
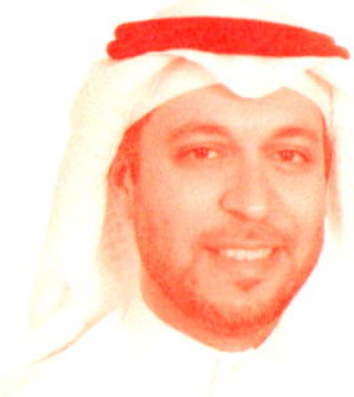
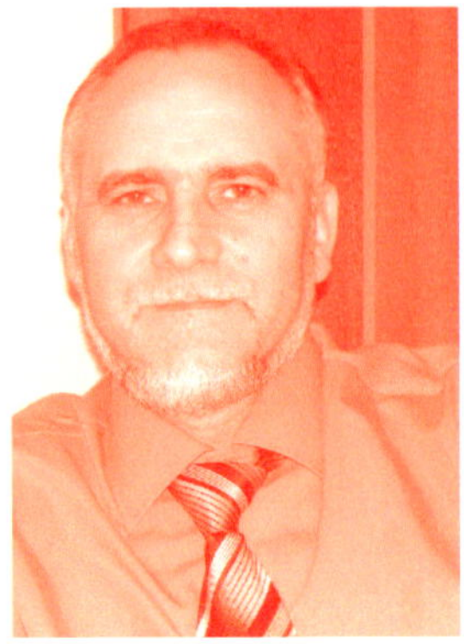
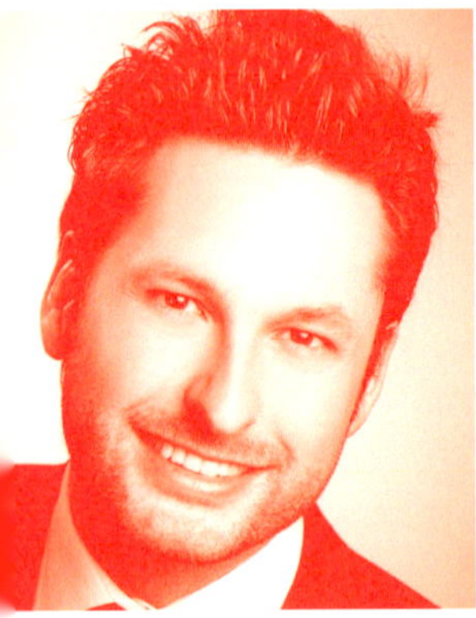
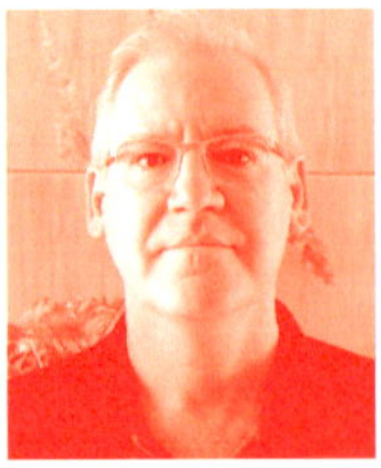
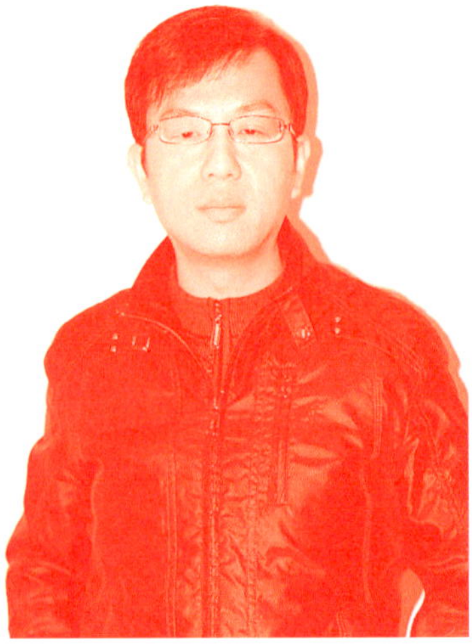

IntechOpen

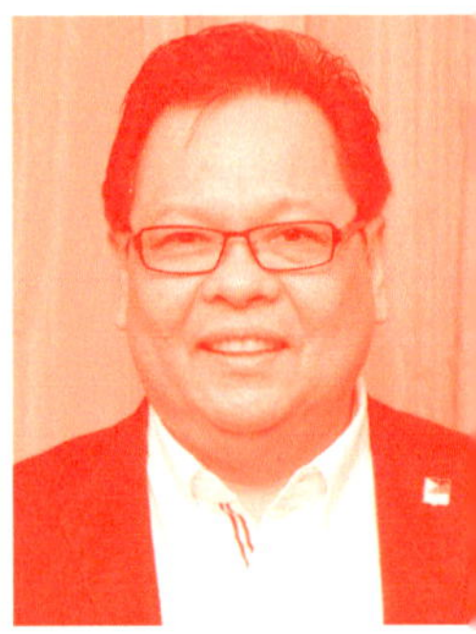
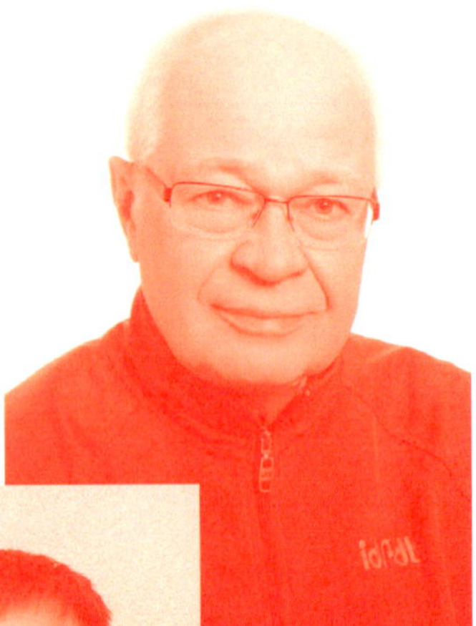
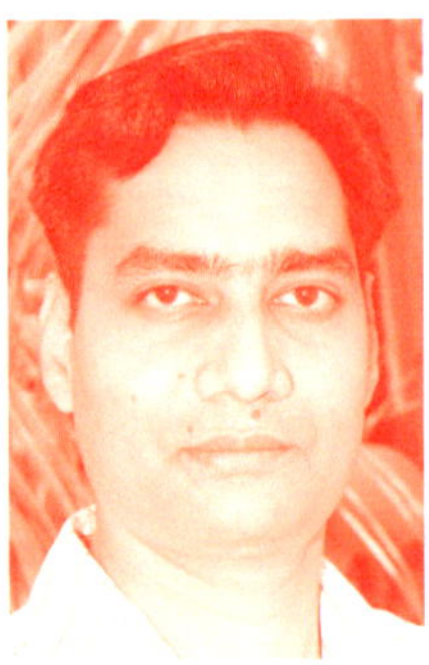
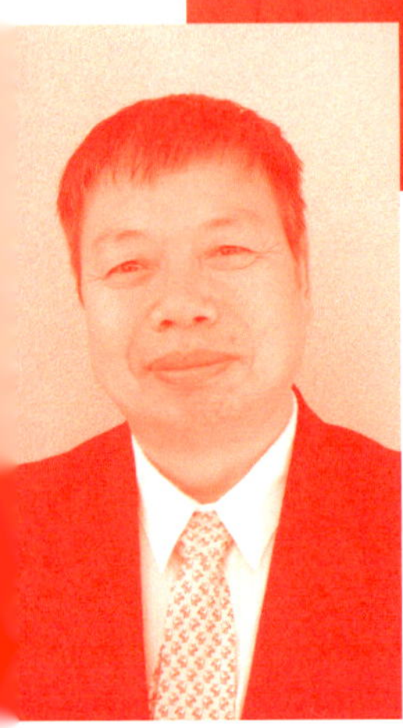
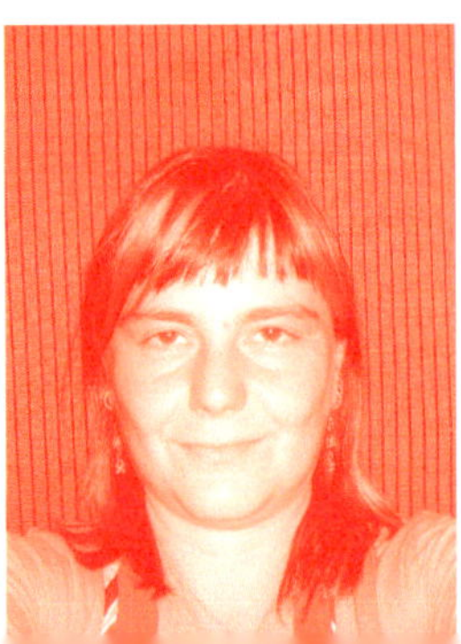
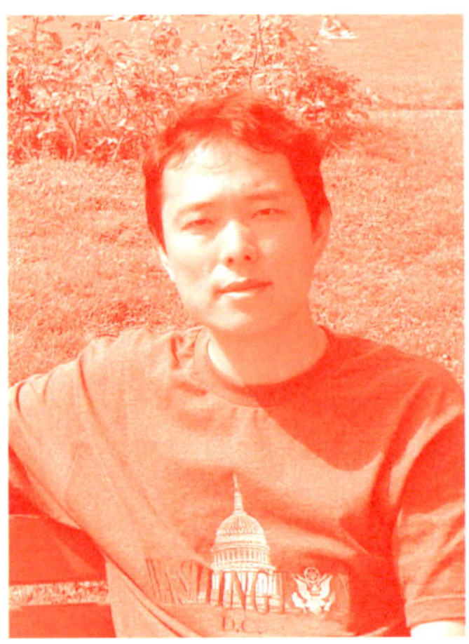

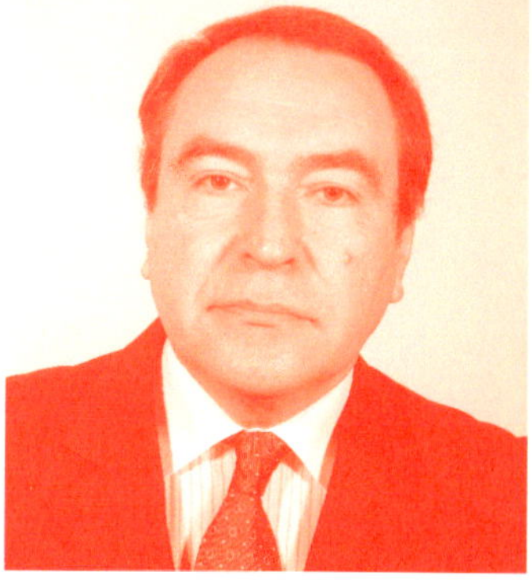
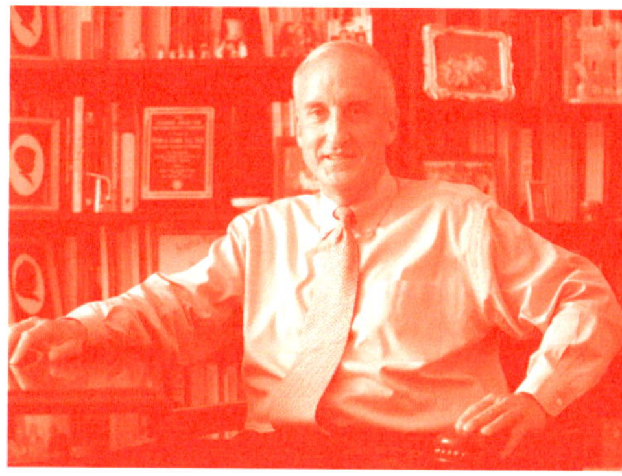
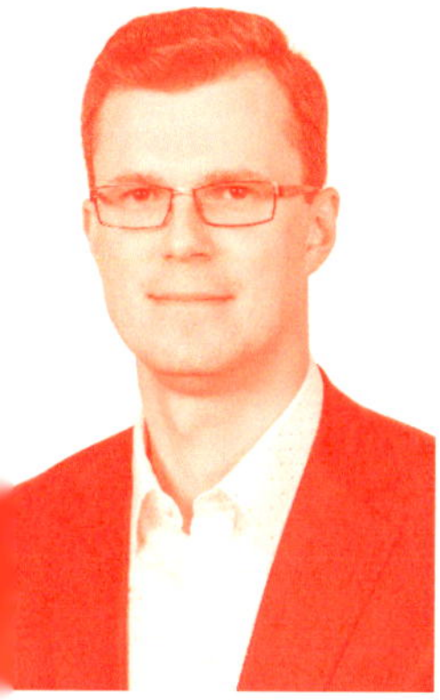
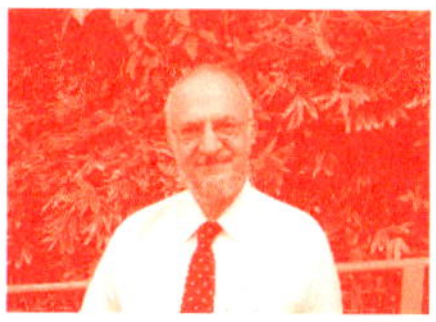
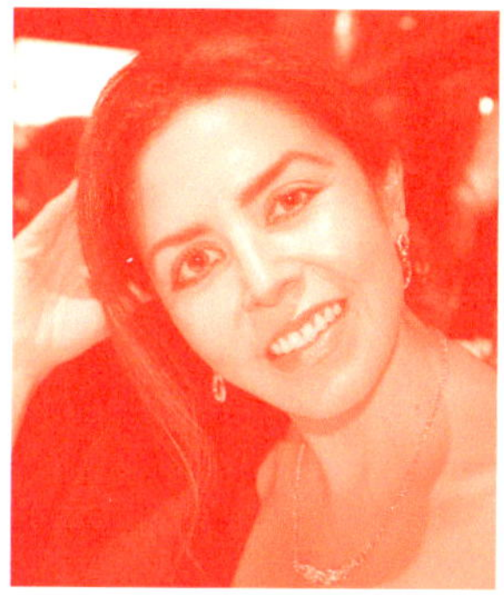

Supporting open minds since 2005

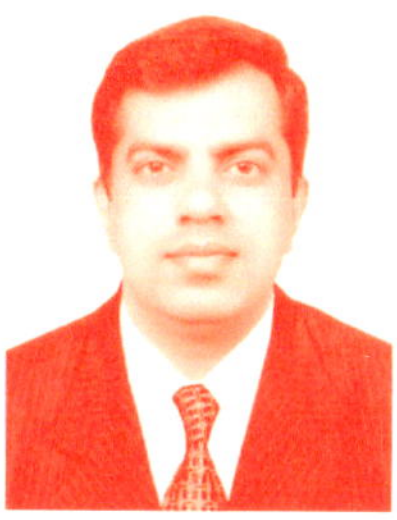
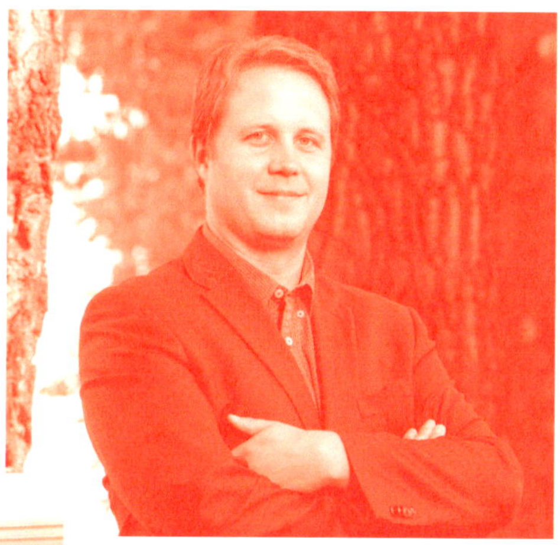
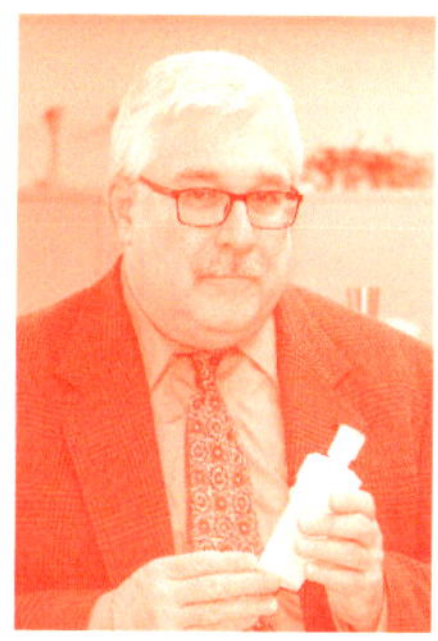
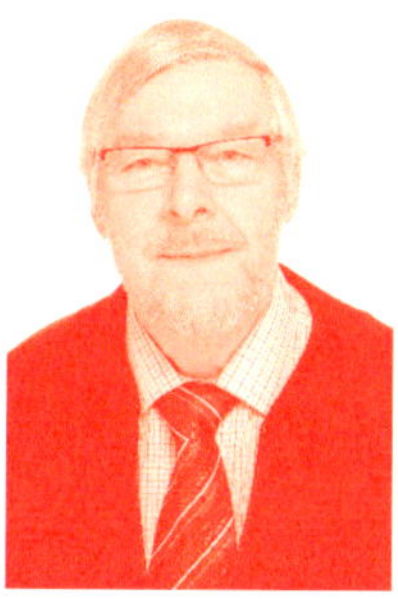
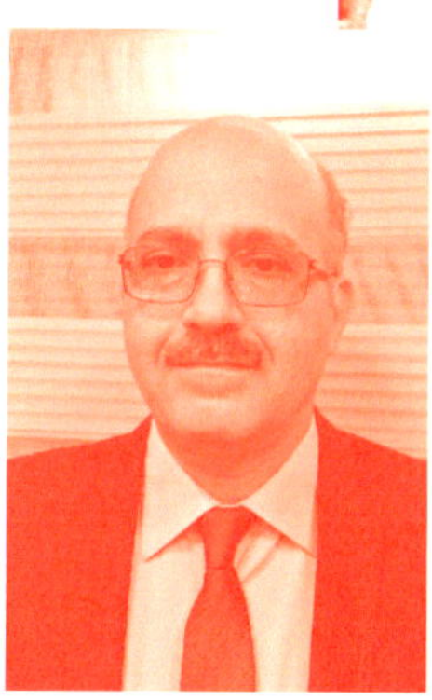
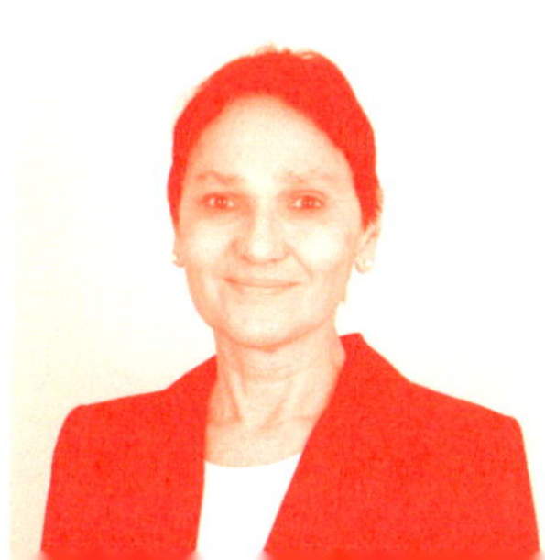
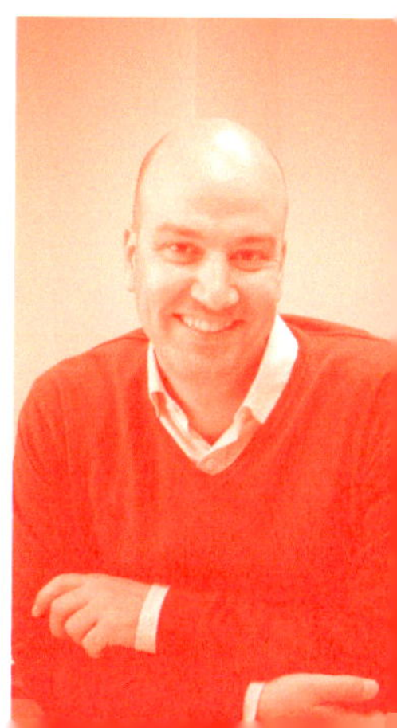

Aortic Aneurysm and Aortic Dissection
http://dx.doi.org/10.5772/intechopen.78173
Edited by Jeffrey Shuhaiber

Contributors
Ruchika Meel, Ricardo Goncalves, Fadi Farhat, Zhenheng Guo, Shu Liu, Ming Gong, Parmanand Singh, Ozan Unlu, Zaid Almarzooq, Matthew Brandorff, Diala Steitieh, Lucas Ribé, Lucía Requejo, Aida Ribes, Manuel Miralles, Mohamed Yacin Sikkandar, Shankar Srinivasan, Abdullah Al Amoudi, Benoit Cosset, Sarah Abdellaoui, Hugo Huvelle, Amine Fikani

First published in London, United Kingdom, 2020 by IntechOpen
IntechOpen is the global imprint of INTECHOPEN LIMITED, registered in England and Wales, registration number: 11086078, 7th floor, 10 Lower Thames Street, London, EC3R 6AF, United Kingdom
Printed in Croatia

British Library Cataloguing-in-Publication Data
A catalogue record for this book is available from the British Library

Additional hard and PDF copies can be obtained from orders@intechopen.com

Aortic Aneurysm and Aortic Dissection
Edited by Jeffrey Shuhaiber
p. cm.
Print ISBN 978-1-78923-977-5
Online ISBN 978-1-78923-978-2
eBook (PDF) ISBN 978-1-83968-395-4

For EU product safety concerns:
IN TECH d.o.o., Prolaz Marije Krucifikse Kozulić 3, 51000 Rijeka, Croatia, info@intechopen.com or visit our website at intechopen.com.

Meet the editor

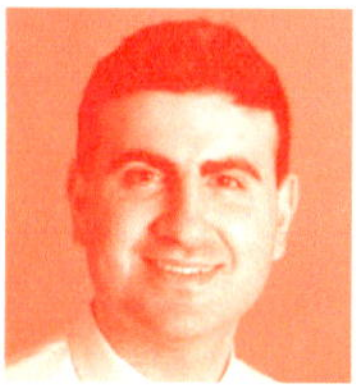

Jeffrey Shuhaiber is a cardiovascular and thoracic surgeon at the Heart and Vascular Center and Department of Surgery at Baystate Medical Center and University of Massachusetts Medical School. Dr. Shuhaiber earned his MD from the University of London King's College School of Medicine with distinction and completed his post-graduate medical education at the same institution. He completed his surgical residency at the University of Illinois and then thoracic surgery at Loyola University, and did his fellowship at Boston Children's Hospital and Cambridge University. He then joined the University of Cincinnati and Children's Hospital as Assistant Professor in Cardiac Surgery. Dr. Shuhaiber has interests in both teaching and clinical research. He has received numerous awards throughout residency and clinical practice. He has had broad training in both acquired and structural heart disease as well as surgery for heart and lung failure. He has been the recipient of first-place awards for research presented at American College of Surgeons Committees. He is a reviewer for several surgical journals and has authored several book chapters, and has authored or coauthored numerous peer-reviewed publications. He performs both clinical and translational research.

Contents

Preface XI

Chapter 1 1
Diagnosis and Surveillance of Aortic Root Dilation
by Ozan Unlu, Zaid I. Almarzooq, Diala Steitieh, Matthew Brandorff and Parmanand Singh

Chapter 2 23
Challenges for Intelligent Data Analysis Methods in Medical Image Analysis during Surgical Interventions of Aneurysms
by Abdullah Al Amoudi, Shankar Srinivasan and Mohamed Yacin Sikkandar

Chapter 3 47
Mycotic Aortic Aneurysms
by Lucas Ribé Bernal, Lucía Requejo, Aida Ribes and Manuel Miralles

Chapter 4 67
Human Immunodeficiency Virus Associated Large Artery Disease
by Ruchika Meel and Ricardo Gonçalves

Chapter 5 77
A New Mouse Model of Aortic Aneurysm Induced by Deoxycorticosterone Acetate or Aldosterone in the Presence of High Salt
by Ming C. Gong, Shu Liu and Zhenheng Guo

Chapter 6 89
Extensive Repair in Type A Aortic Dissection: To Save the Patient or to Ensure a Durable Repair?
by Benoit Cosset, Sarah Abdellaoui, Hugo Huvelle, Amine Fikani and Fadi Farhat

Preface

An aortic aneurysm is an enlargement of the aorta. It is a major global public health problem with unmet needs regarding primary prevention. Aortic aneurysm has an incidence of up to 10 cases per 100,000, and is more common in men older than 60 years. Aortic aneurysm leads to at least 15,000 deaths when it ruptures due to the enlarged aortic wall's weakening. Aneurysm of the aorta can start anywhere from the aortic valve sinuses to the common iliac arteries. Aortic aneurysm etiology remains unknown, yet common cardiovascular risk factors remain strongly associated. Aortic aneurysm mortality has not declined despite our innovations, education, and contributions.

This book reviews the latest information on the diagnosis and surveillance of aortic root dilation, mycotic aortic aneurysm, and the role of human immunodeficiency virus. Written by international experts, chapters discuss such topics as animal models for abdominal aortic aneurysm, safe methods of repairing type A aortic dissection, and challenges in data image analysis. Each chapter is illustrated with tables, figures, and diagrams to enhance content, and contains references for further information. The book provides a simple framework for those who want to understand the principles of aortic aneurysm and aortic dissection repair. It provides a global outlook on the disease and its diagnosis and management.

We hope this book will be of value to all clinicians and healthcare providers as well as patients who want to learn more about aortic aneurysm and aortic dissection. Cardiologists, cardiac surgeons, cardiac pathologists, and radiologists will also learn from this book how to help care for patients with this disease.

Jeffrey Shuhaiber MD
University of Massachusetts,
USA

Chapter 1

Diagnosis and Surveillance of Aortic Root Dilation

Ozan Unlu, Zaid I. Almarzooq, Diala Steitieh, Matthew Brandorff and Parmanand Singh

Abstract

Aortic root dilation (AoD) imparts increased risk of aortic complications such as dissection, rupture, and valvular regurgitation. Multiple etiologies of AoD exist, such as Marfan syndrome, bicuspid aortic valve, Ehler-Danlos syndrome, infections, and idiopathic conditions. Due to the variety of clinical conditions that can result in AoD, and the risks associated with worsening AoD, a thorough understanding of the pathophysiology of AoD, noninvasive imaging modalities, and pharmacologic therapies is critical. This chapter will review the various etiologies of AoD, pathophysiological basis of each disease entity, overview of the diagnosis of AoD, noninvasive imaging modalities employed for detection and surveillance, pharmacological therapies used in the prevention and management, and the factors that guide intervention such as surgical repair.

Keywords: aortic root, enlargement, dilation, aneurysm, noninvasive imaging

1. Introduction

Aortic root dilation (AoD) is frequently an incidentally discovered, asymptomatic finding in that is seen on various imaging modalities [1]. The anatomy of the aortic root includes the annulus, sinuses of Valsalva, sinotubular junction and ascending aorta [1], with the size being a function of a patient's biologic variables such as height, age, BSA, and gender [1, 2]. However, while natural variations in the size of the aortic root are well known, the identification of progression from normal to pathologic AoD is a key clinical diagnosis that carries significant cardiovascular risk including aortic dissection, rupture, valvular regurgitation and cardiac tamponade [1, 3–5]. The etiology of pathological AoD is varied, ranging from congenital, infectious, autoimmune, and idiopathic conditions; and influences the medical and surgical management [1, 5]. Due to the variety of clinical conditions that can result in AoD, and the risks associated with worsening AoD, a thorough understanding of the pathophysiology of AoD, noninvasive imaging modalities and pharmacologic therapies is critical. The aim of this chapter is to review the most common conditions associated with AoD, appropriate imaging modalities, and treatment strategies to manage AoD.

2. Etiologies of aortic root dilation

Multiple etiologies of AoD exist such as Marfan syndrome, bicuspid aortic valve, Loeys-Dietz and Ehler-Danlos syndromes, idiopathic conditions, hypertension, infections, and inflammatory disorders. In this chapter, we will discuss the various etiologies categorized into two standardized groups—genetically-mediated and nongenetically mediated AoD.

2.1 Genetically-mediated aortic root dilation

Genetically-mediated aortic root dilation or enlargement is the leading cause of thoracic aortic aneurysms. Marfan syndrome (MFS), the prototype condition for AoD, and bicuspid aortic valve has led to a greater understanding of AoD pathophysiology, pharmacologic treatment, timing of surgical intervention and optimal surveillance strategies with noninvasive imaging [6].

2.1.1 Marfan syndrome

MFS is one of the most common hereditary disorders of connective tissues and is characterized by manifestations in cardiovascular, skeletal, and ocular systems [7]. MFS is the most common genetic cause of thoracic aortic aneurysms (TAAs). Its inheritance is almost exclusively autosomal dominant and mostly involves a mutation of the fibrillin-1 (FBN1) gene encoding the connective tissue structural protein fibrillin-1 [8]. The widely accepted incidence of Marfan syndrome is ~1 in 5000 individuals [9].

Although the inheritance pattern is predominantly autosomal dominant, rare cases of autosomal recessive FBN1 gene mutations has been described [10]. While patients with Marfan phenotypes usually have an affected family member, 25% of the cases are sporadic due to *de novo* mutations [9]. In addition, in <10% of Marfan cases, no mutation of FBN1 was determined [11]. Since it was first identified as the main cause of Marfan syndrome, FBN1 mutations, depending on how it is mutated, were linked to a variety of syndromes and phenotypes [12]. Animal studies investigating the pathophysiology of the disease demonstrated overexpression of TGF-β in the mitral valve preceding prolapse, the aorta associated with dilatation, skeletal muscle associated with myopathy, and the dura leading to ectasia [12]. Later, mutations in TGF-beta receptor 2 (TGFBR2) and TGFBR1 genes were identified in some patients with Marfan phenotypes and subsequently implicated in the disease process in FBN1 mutation negative individuals [13–15]. These genes were also linked to another condition later, namely Loeys-Dietz syndrome (LDS) [14].

The diagnosis of Marfan syndrome is established by using a combination of clinical manifestations, family history, and the presence of FBN1 mutation. In order to facilitate accurate recognition of the syndrome and improve patient management and counseling, a set of defined clinical criteria, called the Ghent nosology was developed [16] and later revised [17] (**Table 1**). Apart from the genetic testing for FBN1 mutation, Ghent nosology uses a systemic score calculation using clinical manifestations of Marfan and an aortic root dilatation Z-score (see noninvasive imaging below).

One of the major causes of mortality and clinical hallmark of Marfan syndrome is aortic root dilation and related complications such as dissection, rupture and/or aortic valvular regurgitation. Aortic root dilation is typically first identified on echocardiography in 60–80% of Marfan patients [18]. Therefore, surveillance echocardiography has been routinely used to serially monitor aortic dimensions. If the aortic root diameter is above 4.5 cm in adults, aortic dilation rates are above 0.5 cm/year, and/or significant aortic insufficiency is already present, more frequent monitoring is recommended [6] (see Diagnosis and Surveillance of Aortic Root Dilation below for more detailed guidelines).

DOI: http://dx.doi.org/10.5772/intechopen.86329

Patients with family history of Marfan disease
• Ectopia lentis
• Systemic score ≥ 7
• Aortic root dilatation Z-score ≥2 in patients above 20 years old ≥2 in patients below 20 years old
Patients without family history of Marfan disease
• Aortic root dilatation Z-score ≥ 2 and Ectopia lentis
• Aortic root dilatation Z-score ≥ 2 and FBN1 mutation
• Aortic root dilatation Z-score ≥ 2 and systemic score ≥ 7
• Ectopia lentis and FBN1 mutation associated with aortic root dilatation

Table 1.
Revised Ghent nosology.

2.1.2 Bicuspid aortic valve

Bicuspid aortic valve is one of the most frequent congenital heart anomalies in adults, affecting 0.9–2% of the population [19]. Most cases of bicuspid aortic valve are familial and studies show that heritability of the disease is ~90% making it an autosomal dominant pattern with incomplete penetrance [20]. Bicuspid aortic valve can occur alone or with other congenital cardiovascular disorders such as coarctation of the aorta, supravalvular or subvalvular aortic stenosis, and ventricular septal defect [21].

The diagnosis is often established by transthoracic echocardiogram (TTE), which has high sensitivity (~92%) and specificity (~96%) [22]. TTE is also useful for surveillance of potential complications of bicuspid aorta such as aortic stenosis, aortic dilation, aortic regurgitation, and infective endocarditis [23]. Given the risk of inheritance, first degree relatives are also recommended to be screened with TTE [21].

Prevalence of aortic dilation in patients with bicuspid aortic valve disease ranges from 20 to 84% depending on the criteria used in different studies [24]. The risk of aortic dilation increases with age and the risk of dissection increases as the aortic diameter increases [25, 26]. When the aortic root diameter is above 4.5 cm, there is a family history of aortic dissection, or aortic diameter change is rapid it is recommended to perform echocardiogram annually [21]. More frequent surveillance is recommended for patients with aortic root diameters approaching surgical thresholds (see Surgical Interventions section below).

2.1.3 Loeys-Dietz syndrome

Loeys-Dietz syndrome (LDS) is a rare congenital syndrome characterized by hypertelorism (widely spaced eyes), a split uvula or cleft palate, tortuous arteries and aortic aneurysms. LDS shares many features with Marfan syndrome [14]. Most of the LDS cases are sporadic or show an autosomal dominant pattern of inheritance [14].

The incidence and prevalence of the disease is still not well established.

Loeys-Dietz syndrome was initially classified into two subtypes based on the severity of the cutaneous and craniofacial features but later was divided into six subtypes stratified by genotypes [27]. These subtypes are labeled 1–6 and associated with mutations in TGFBR1, TGFBR2, SMAD3, TGFB2, TGFB3, SMAD2, respectively [27]. Type 1 and type 2 are the most commonly seen subtypes with frequencies of 20 and 55% among all subtypes, respectively [28].

Aortic root dilation is a hallmark feature of this disease entity and is frequently seen in patients (~80%) [29]. Another vascular manifestation is aneurysms throughout the arterial tree. This is a concerning clinical manifestations of the disease and can cause aggressive arteriopathy; therefore, early operative intervention at ascending aortic diameters of ≥42 mm is recommended [30].

2.1.4 Ehler-Danlos syndrome

Ehlers-Danlos syndromes (EDS) are a heterogeneous and relatively rare group of connective tissue disorders characterized by skin hyperextensibility, joint hypermobility, and tissue fragility [31]. Ehler-Danlos syndrome can present with a variety of clinical manifestations and can be caused by different kinds of genetic mutations. Overall prevalence of EDS is ~1 in 5000 and EDS hypermobile (hEDS) is the most common type [31].

Vascular complications can be seen with different types of EDS; however, it is most commonly seen in type IV (vascular or arterial ecchymotic type; vESD), characterized by an autosomal dominant mutation in COL3A1 (collagen, type III, α-1 gene) encoding type III procollagen [32]. Up to 80% with vESD patients suffer from vascular complications by the age 40 years [32]. Therefore EDS patients, especially vEDS, patients should be routinely evaluated for aortic root disease. These patients are recommended to undergo elective operation at smaller diameters (4.0–5.0 cm) to avoid acute dissection or rupture. Patients with a growth rate of more than 0.5 cm/year in an aorta that is <5.5 cm in diameter are recommended to be considered for operation [33].

2.2 Nongenetic

2.2.1 Idiopathic

Aortic root dilation is an established phenomenon that has shown strong correlations to key pathobiological factors such as age, body surface area (BSA), height and gender. The correlation of aortic root size with age and BSA were initially described in the development of screening nomograms using M-mode echocardiograms [34]. Follow up studies with 2D echocardiography further validated these correlations, allowing for the development of nomograms for normal patient populations or adjusted for patients with underlying congenital disorders (i.e., Marfan syndrome) [2, 35]. These studies evaluating AoD by echocardiograms are further supported by reviews of autopsy data that show clear correlations to key pathobiological factors such as increased age and height with AoD [36].

Despite the validation of age as being correlated strongly with AoD, the mechanism of age on the development of AoD still remains an area of active research. One of the predominant hypotheses is based on the idea of cyclic stress, and how the aorta degrades through gradual mechanical decline of elastin proteins [37]. Elastic arteries, namely the aorta, are estimated to dilate by 10% with each beat [38]. It is hypothesized that the shear stress over a normal lifetime results in the degradation of elastic lamella, resulting in arterial dilation and stiffening [38]. This is corroborated by histologic data demonstrating damage to medial elastin of the proximal aorta [38]. Furthermore, there is evidence to suggest that in the absence of risk factors such as hypertension or atherosclerosis, the aortic wall undergoes age-associated reprograming that is proinflammatory promotes progression of arterial disease [39]. Wang et al. demonstrated in pathologic samples of aortas that age correlated with increased smooth muscle cell invasion, and increased production of downstream angiotensin II mediators [39].

In addition to age and BSA, gender is another key factor which can increase the risk and progression of AoD [40]. In the Framingham study of 1849 men and 2152 women, not currently diagnosed with cardiac disease or having a cardiac history, aortic root was 2.4 mm smaller in women than men with m-mode echocardiography [40]. A systematic review in 2014 of 10,741 patients with hypertension revealed men had a significantly higher incidence of AoD relative to women [41].

In conclusion, a series of biological variables are correlated with AoD, and it is important to take these into account as they are potential confounders or contributors in the evaluation of patients with pathologic AoD. Even exercise capacity has been correlated with AoD, with a recent meta-analysis showing that athletes defined by participation in National Collegiate Athletic Association (NCAA) or international equivalent had an aortic root diameter that was larger than nonathletic controls [42], and a statistically significant increase by measurement of sinuses of Valsalva and aortic root annulus [42]. It is important to understand the significance of biological variables such as age, height, BSA, or gender to fully evaluate pathologic AoD without the influence of known confounders.

2.2.2 HTN

Hypertension is a well-known risk factor for aortic dissection, and in some studies, it is estimated to factor into roughly half of the overall risk for aortic dissection [43]. A recent prospective cohort study of 30,447 patients, 86% of patients who developed aortic dissection had hypertension [4]. However the relationship between hypertension and AoD is not as clearly established. In a Framingham study of 3195 patients, there was no relationship between the development of AoD with hypertension [44]. A subsequent follow up study of Framingham participants evaluating aortic root diameter was positively correlated with mean arterial pressure, but negatively associated with pulse pressure, indicating that the mechanism behind AoD is more complicated [45]. Moreover, investigations have shown that in patients with other comorbidities for AoD, such as, Turner syndrome, hypertension is significantly associated with increased prevalence of AoD [45]. This has led to interesting insights into the cyclic stress hypothesis of the development of AoD [43]. If AoD develops due to chronic shear stress, then it would be expected that AoD is correlated with higher pulse pressure (PP), which would presumably lead to greater stress and aortic dilation [43]. However, studies have reported an inverse relationship between AoD and PP [43]. Additionally a systematic review in 2014 showed that in a population of 10,791 hypertensive patients, 9.1% had AoD with a significant gender skew toward men [41]. However there was no significant correlation of mean arterial pressure or pulse pressure values and AoD [41]. While hypertensive patients have a higher incidence of AoD, the mechanism remains to be further investigated. Moreover, these unclear correlations between MAP, PP, and AoD suggest that the aorta is not static, but a dynamic structure whose response to stress, such as hypertension, is still being elucidated [43].

2.2.3 Infections

Since the first mass production of penicillin in 1945, the modern era of antibiotics has resulted in a decrease in the prevalence of mycotic aneurysms due to bacterial infections in developed countries [46, 47]. However they can still be found in developing countries, and are rare but well described causes of mycotic aneurysms [46]. Most common pathogens include *Salmonella*, *Staphylococcus* and *Streptococcus pneumonia*, and while rare have been in the pathogenesis of mycotic aneurysms of the aortic root [46, 48, 49]. Other common bacteria include *Mycobacterium tuberculosis* and *Treponema pallidum*, which will be discussed below, and more rare causes include *Listeria*, *Bacteroides*, *Clostridium septicum*, and *Campylobacter jejuni* [46]. With the majority of bacterial aortitis, aneurysm development is generally saccular, and *Salmonella* has been reported in case studies to predominantly affect the abdominal aorta than the thoracic [46, 48]. Infections with Staphylococcal species generally are related to underlying aortic valve infections, but have been reported to progress into aneurysms of the aortic root [46, 49].

2.2.3.1 *Treponema pallidum*

Treponema pallidum, a sexually transmitted spirochete which is the causative organism of syphilis, is a well characterized cause of aortitis [46, 50, 51]. Cardiovascular involvement is limited to late stage, or tertiary syphilis, and generally occurs 5 to upwards of 40 years after primary infection [50, 51]. Aortitis, and aneurysm development is due to invasion of the vasa vasorum, resulting in obliterative endarteritis that leads to degradation of the aortic media [50, 51]. The chronic inflammation results in fibrosis of the intima, a phenomenon known as "tree-barking" that ultimately progresses to aneurysm development. In an autopsy study in 1960 of 51 aortic aneurysms secondary to syphilitic aortitis, 7.8% were found at the sinuses of Valsalva and 29.4% involved the ascending aorta, representing a majority of the sample [52]. This predominance to the ascending thoracic aorta have been further corroborated in later studies, however the detailed echocardiographic analysis of syphilitic aortitis, specifically in relation to AoD is limited due to the rarity of the disease presentation [46, 50].

2.2.3.2 *Tuberculosis*

Tuberculosis is a relatively common infection especially in developing countries [53]. *Mycobacterium tuberculosis*, the causative pathogen, is a known cause of mycotic aortic aneurysms [46, 50]. Pathogenesis of tuberculous mycotic aneurysm is believed to be due to lymphatic spread or hematogenous seeding, and mortality rates are reported as high as 60% in patients who develop this complication [50]. While more commonly affecting the distal aortic arch and descending aorta, there are case reports detailing aortic root aneurysms due to tuberculosis [50, 54].

2.2.3.3 *HIV*

There have been case reports proposing an association between aortic aneurysms and HIV [50]. In a variety of these cases the causes are generally multifactorial, as the majority of cases have reported coinfections (Q fever and leishmaniasis) or comorbid autoimmune conditions (giant cell arteritis) [55, 56]. It is still an area of investigation as to whether there is a true association, and there is sparse data showing a relationship with AoD.

2.2.4 *Inflammatory disorders*

2.2.4.1 *Ankylosing spondylitis*

Ankylosing spondylitis, a seronegative spondyloarthropathy, is a chronic, progressive rheumatologic disorder, and was one of the first found to be associated with aortitis [50, 57]. The proposed mechanism of AoD in ankylosing spondylitis is fibrous growth development along the intima, which leads to subsequent weakening [57]. Prior TEE studies further evaluated the prevalence of AoD in ankylosing spondylitis, and 82% of patients with ankylosing spondylitis had aortic root abnormalities [58]. Specifically, 61% of patients had aortic root thickening and 25% of patients had AoD [58]. AoD in these populations is a relatively common phenomenon and is associated with significant cardiac morbidity [45, 57].

2.2.4.2 Relapsing polychondritis

Relapsing polychondritis is another autoimmune disorder, which is a multisystem inflammatory disorder that primarily affects the cartilaginous structures of the body [59]. Cardiovascular involvement is common, estimated to be the second most frequent cause of death and can result in aneurysm development in 5% of cases of both thoracic and abdominal aorta [50, 59]. AoD has been known to occur, albeit rare, with cases of requiring surgical revision after the development of aortic regurgitation [60, 61].

2.2.4.3 Takayasu arteritis

Takayasu arteritis is a chronic granulomatous large vessel vasculitis, predominantly found in pediatric populations [50, 62]. A rare disorder, the pathogenesis is characterized by granulomatous panarteritis that can affect the entirety of the aorta and major branches, however predominantly affects the common carotid and subclavian artery [62]. While rare, there are reports of AoD from Takayasu arteritis resulting in aortic regurgitation [63, 64].

2.2.4.4 Giant cell arteritis

Giant cell arteritis is a large vessel vasculitis that is characterized by chronic granulomatous inflammation [50]. While commonly affecting carotid, temporal and vertebral arteries, it has been known to affect the ascending aorta, at times resulting in dissection or aortic valve insufficiency [50]. The development of AoD from GCA may be influenced by other comorbid conditions such as HIV; however, this association is currently only supported with case reports [55].

2.2.5 Other

2.2.5.1 Left ventricular hypertrophy

Additionally left ventricular hypertrophy is reported to be positively correlated with AoD. Early retrospective reviews of echocardiographic studies have shown a positive relationship between LVH and AoD, and this has been further supported in subsequent systematic reviews [41, 65]. Patients with AoD with concomitant left ventricular hypertrophy are shown to have an increased risk of adjusted cardiovascular events [66]. However as with previous studies, the exact mechanism between LVH and AoD is still being determined.

3. Diagnosis and surveillance of aortic dilation

3.1 Clinical manifestations

Aortic root dilation is typically a silent disease, with most cases being diagnosed incidentally on imaging. AoD can become symptomatic as the aneurysm enlarges. Aortic root aneurysms grow at an average of 1–4 mm/year [5], with a faster rate of growth noted in patients with bicuspid aortic valves, Marfan syndrome, ESRD, male gender, and smokers [5, 67]. When the aneurysm enlarges to the point of compressing surrounding structures the patient may begin to observe symptoms—the most common of which is chest pain, seen in up to 75% of patients [5, 68]. Other nonspecific symptoms can include back pain, abdominal pain and fatigue (though only present in 5% of patients).

Additionally, patients may present with symptoms secondary to complications of a dilated aortic root such as aortic insufficiency and congestive heart failure. Thus, patients can develop dyspnea as the presenting symptom of aortic root dilation up to 40% of the time [68]. Other presenting symptoms may be related to the complications noted in **Table 2** [69–74].

3.1.1 Complications of aortic root dilation

Acute aortic emergencies that occur secondary to aortic root dilation include dissection, rupture, and aortic insufficiency. As the aortic root diameter increases, the risk for aortic dissection and rupture rises [75]. Aortic dissections are the most common acute aortic emergencies [76], and can be classified depending on the segment of the aorta affected: type A dissections involve the ascending aorta (seen in aortic root dilation), while type B dissections are those that occur distal to the left subclavian artery.

Aortic dissection most commonly presents with acute onset chest pain that may radiate to the back. The character of the pain has traditionally been described as ripping or tearing in nature, however over half of patients may instead complain of sharp pain [77]. In addition, geriatric populations are less likely to have an acute onset of pain [78]. Physical exam findings that may be present include unequal blood pressures in the upper extremities, a new diastolic murmur indicative of acute aortic regurgitation, or muffled heart sounds secondary to tamponade (with proximal extension of the dissection). Imaging may be notable for widening of the mediastinum on CXR [77]. In order to aid in the diagnosis of a dissection, an aortic dissection detection risk score (ADD-RS) has been developed. The score is comprised of three categories: the presence of high risk conditions such as Marfan syndrome, the presence of typical symptoms (such as abrupt onset chest pain), and the presence of physical exam findings such as unequal blood pressure readings in the upper extremities. Each group is given a score of 1 if a feature is present, and the total score helps pave the next steps of workup—a score of 0 can be followed by diagnostic workup of other pathologies, while scores of 2–3 should be followed by expedited workup and immediate surgical consultation for possible aortic dissection [79].

Complication of aortic root aneurysm	Presenting symptom
Aortic insufficiency, aortic regurgitation	Dyspnea, diastolic murmur, congestive heart failure symptoms
Aortic dissection	Sharp chest pain, may radiate to the back
Thromboembolism	Symptoms of stroke
Compression of tracheal or bronchus	Hemoptysis, cough, recurrent pneumonitis
Compression of left recurrent laryngeal nerve	Hoarseness
Compression of superior vena cava	Signs of superior vena cava syndrome
Compression of esophagus	Dysphagia

Table 2.
Complications and presenting symptoms of aortic root dilation.

Aortic rupture is also an acute and life-threatening complication of aortic root dilation. It can present similarly to aortic dissection with regards to chest pain, however rupture can lead to severe and abrupt hypotension. Moreover, contingent with the site of rupture the patient may have symptoms such as hemoptysis [80] (if there is rupture into the lung), hematemesis [81] (if there is rupture into the esophagus), or cardiogenic shock [82] (if there is rupture into the pericardial cavity with resultant tamponade physiology).

Aortic root dilation may also lead to aortic insufficiency. Roughly 30% of aortic insufficiency is now recognized as being caused by aortic root dilation, surpassing the incidence of any valvular cause [83]. The pathophysiology is related to stretching of the aortic valve annulus secondary to aortic root dilation, which results in incomplete closure of the aortic leaflets during diastole. Unfortunately, at the onset of aortic regurgitation, patients may be asymptomatic; therefore, congestive heart failure can develop when the regurgitant valve goes unnoticed.

3.1.2 Impact/burden on public health

While aortic root aneurysms are known to grow at an average of 1–4 mm/year [5], it is difficult to ascertain how fast an individual's aortic root aneurysm will grow, therefore necessitating surveillance imaging. The frequency of surveillance imaging recommended is dependent on the etiology of the aortic root dilatation as well as its size, with genetically mediated aortic disease having a lower threshold for more frequent (biannual) imaging [84]. At the very least however patients are recommended to have annual imaging for aortic root dilation to closely monitor the aortic diameter. The impact that frequent imaging (CT, MR angiography or echocardiography) has on public health is likely significant, with cumulative costs. In addition, any patient with a bicuspid aortic valve should be screened for a thoracic aortic aneurysm, as well as screening all first-degree family members of a patient with genetic conditions such as Marfan syndrome [85].

3.2 Noninvasive imaging

The aortic root is the most proximal segment of the aorta. It extends from the annulus of the aortic valve to the sinotubular junction (STJ). It is composed of the left, right, and non coronary sinuses of Valsalva. The diameter of the aorta decreases as it moves distally. The aortic root is assessed using multimodality imaging techniques. These include transthoracic echocardiogram (TTE), cardiac magnetic resonance imaging (cMRI), and cardiac computed tomography angiography (cCTA).

3.2.1 Transthoracic echocardiogram

TTE is widely used for the detection and monitoring of aortic root pathology. Early studies established age- and sex-specific nomograms for aortic root measurements [86]. These studies used the motion mode (M-mode) of TTE, in which the amplitude of the ultrasound pulses amplitudes is converted to corresponding level on gray-scale imaging [86]. Using the M-mode, the American Society of Echocardiography (ASE) has recommended using the leading-edge to leading-edge approach for measuring the aortic root [87]. Later studies used 2D TTE and obtained reference measurements of the aortic root. This is now preferred over M-mode images, which may be off-axis and are subject to aortic motion that may produce erroneous measurements.

On echocardiogram, the aortic root diameter is typically measured in the parasternal long-axis view from the right coronary sinus to the opposite sinus of Valsalva. When unable to obtain the long axis view, the parasternal short axis view may provide more accurate measurements. However, universal landmarks to measure the root in this view have not been established. Some suggest measuring the diameter from the right coronary sinus to the opposite commissure. These measurements are typically performed at end diastole, as this represents the resting aortic diameter [88]. In adults, these measurements correlate with age and body size. In addition, the aorta is about 2 mm larger in men compared to women due to differences in body size [89]. Normal values stratified by body surface area and age have been published by the ASE [87].

Importantly, TTE is limited by its two-dimensional images and thus does not give a complete depiction of the aortic root. It is also limited by patient factors that limit the visualization windows and thus aortic root measurement. Since the aorta is not a straight tube, it can be imaged obliquely leading to over-estimation of its true diameter. Newer modalities, such cMRI and cCTA, can provide three-dimensional images.

3.2.2 Cardiac magnetic resonance imaging

Despite ECG-gated CT being the most accurate modality for evaluating the thoracic aorta, it is limited by the radiation and contrast exposure. This is particularly important in younger patients with connective tissue disorders that require serial follow up imaging. Cardiac MRI provides an alternative approach for imaging the thoracic aorta including the aortic root and is considered the preferred modality in select groups. It can be performed with ECG gating to provide motion-free evaluation of the aorta. In addition, young patients, in whom this is more commonly used, can hold their breath for longer periods, allowing acquisition of images with high spatial resolution.

Cardiac MRI evaluation of the aorta does not require contrast use. MRI sequences used include balanced steady-state free precession (SSFP) sequences, fast imaging employing steady-state acquisition (FIESTA), true fast imaging with steady-state precession (FISP), and balanced fast-field echo (FFE) sequences. These sequences provide a high signal-to-noise ratio and adequate contrast between vessel wall and blood pool [90]. When used with ECG gating and contrast enhanced MRA, images tend to have less artifact, higher resolution, and overall short imaging time. Another approach is to use ECG gating 2D balanced SSFP sequence that is oriented perpendicular to the aortic root in two planes to assess the aortic valve and root throughout the cardiac cycle. In addition, prospective ECG gating and respiratory navigation with three-dimensional balanced SSFP sequences can provide 3D aortic imaging without contrast administration [91, 92].

It is important to note that different methods of aortic measurement have been described and guidelines are less well defined. Aortic root measurements can be challenging given different approaches. Burman et al. found in the Framingham Heart Study that cusp-commissure dimensions better corresponded with reference echocardiographic aortic root measurements [89, 93]. This best correlated with study measurements after averaging the three end-diastolic cusp-commissure measurements [93]. In addition, there is a lack of consensus with regard to measurements used (inner lumen only versus lumen and wall) and whether measurements should be adjusted to body surface area, sex, and age.

3.2.3 Cardiac computed tomography

Although TTE is widely used for the imaging and surveillance of aortic root, cardiac computed tomography angiography (cCTA) is currently the most commonly used technique for the study of the thoracic aorta. Main advantages of cCTA are fast scanning times, low artifact sensibility, and wide availability including emergency rooms operating 24 h [94].

The new generation CT scanners acquire high-resolution 3D datasets of the thoracic aorta, showing sensitivities up to 100% and specificities of 98–99% [95]. ECG synchronization is vital for detailed assessment of the aortic root anatomy since it allows suppression of pulsation artifacts [96]. ECG gating also allows viewing images in a particular phase of the cardiac cycle. Unfortunately, the ECG-gated technique can increase the acquisition time and required breath-hold time. In order to minimize the increased acquisition times, employment of a 64 or wider ECG-gated row detector system is suggested [95, 97].

Modern CT scanners can be used to employ several different cardiac synchronization methods such as prospective ECG triggering where images are only acquired during a specified portion of the cardiac cycle, starting at a predetermined delay from the R wave; retrospective ECG gating where the desired cardiac phase is selected retrospectively from the raw data [95, 97]. The details of each technique will not be discussed in this chapter; however, it is important to determine the advantages and disadvantages of different techniques. The main limitations of CT are related to the radiation exposure and the use of iodinated contrast media and different techniques come at a higher cost of each limitation.

For the surveillance of aortic root, any technique can be used and be useful; therefore, the technique with the least amount of radiation exposure should be selected such as prospective sequential triggering without padding, retrospective gating with tube-current modulation optimized for diastolic-phase datasets only, or a prospectively triggered high-pitch helical acquisition [95, 97]. Retrospective ECG gating acquires redundant helical CT data which allows the reconstruction of images at different cardiac phases and providing detailed images which can be useful in complicated cases and pre-/post-operative imaging since pseudoaneurysm or small leaks which are some of the most common complications of aortic root surgery can only be detected during a specific phase of the cardiac cycle. Iodinated contrast-media is another risk related to CT imaging given the risk of contrast induced nephropathy and allergic reactions of various severity. Surveillance CT data for the dimensions of aortic root can be acquired without contrast injection; however, a complete endoluminal evaluation can only be achieved by the injection of contrast-medium [97].

It is standard of care to monitor the size of aortic aneurysms that are below surgical threshold, <5.5 cm for nongenetic aneurysms and <5.0 cm for genetically-mediated aneurysms [98]. In general, physicians should be conscientious about patient cumulative radiation exposure as there is evidence that it can increase cancer incidence and cancer mortality [99]. One study estimated that ionizing radiation exposure results in 0.7% of total expected baseline cancer incidence and 1% of total cancer mortality. These rates increase with greater cumulative exposure [99]. Therefore, physicians should opt to perform serial CT imaging with longer intervals in the most appropriate patients. A study investigating patients with moderate-risk thoracic aortic aneurysms (defined as size <5.0 cm) showed that patients with aneurysms below 4.3 cm had overall lower risk of significant aneurysm growth or size reaching surgical threshold. Thus, the authors suggested that these subset of patients undergo surveillance CT scans less frequently.

4. Management and prevention of aortic root dilation

Management focuses on slowing the rate of growth and the complications of aortic root dilation. The line of management that is chosen for a patient depends on symptoms and size of the aneurysm. For patients who are asymptomatic and have root dilation <55 mm, medical management is advised. In patients with Marfan syndrome or a bicuspid aortic valve, the cut off of ≤50 mm is used for medical management [1, 100].

4.1 Medical management

4.1.1 Beta blockers

The use of beta blockers has shown a survival benefit in patients with aortic root dilation secondary to Marfan syndrome [101]. While data on survival benefits for patients with bicuspid aortic valves is sparse, the common practice is to also prescribe beta blockers given that both conditions share a similar pathology and therefore both are likely to benefit from beta blockade. The mechanism by which beta blockers slow the progression of aortic root dilation is through their negative inotropic and chronotropic effects, reducing the peak left ventricular ejection rate and therefore decreasing shear stress and the rate of aortic dilation [102].

4.1.2 Other agents for blood pressure control

The goal blood pressure for patients with thoracic aortic aneurysms is <130/80 mmHg. In patients who cannot tolerate beta blockers, calcium channel blockers (CCB) are an alternative group of medications available. While less studied as compared to beta blockers, CCB have also been found to reduce the rate of aortic root dilation [103]. Other agents that can be used for additional blood pressure control include ACE-inhibitors and ARBs.

4.1.3 Management of other cardiovascular risk factors

In order to reduce the risk for complications such as aortic dissection, patients should be counseled on smoking cessation, and cessation of drugs that increase aortic wall stress such as cocaine or other stimulants. In addition patients should have dyslipidemia well controlled, which can be achieved through the use of atorvastatin 40–80 mg daily in individuals with aortic root aneurysms [104, 105].

4.1.4 Lifestyle modifications and pregnancy

Patients should be counseled on avoiding high intensity and collision sports, such as boxing and cycling. Instead patients should take part in low dynamic sports, such as, golf [5, 106]. Pregnancy should be avoided in patients with Marfan syndrome with an aortic diameter >40 mm, if a patient does chose to become pregnant however there must be close follow up with surveillance imaging of the aortic diameter [5, 101].

4.2 Surgical management

4.2.1 Indications for surgery

Emergent surgical interventions are indicated for management of an aortic dissection or rupture, or a symptomatic aneurysm. In addition, surgical repair can be performed electively in high risk patients to prevent propagation of an aneurysm (**Table 3**). Indications for elective surgical intervention include the absolute size of the aneurysm—if the diameter is over 55 mm, or over 50 mm in patients with Marfan syndrome or bicuspid valves. Other indications for elective surgery include if the rate

Emergent surgical repair	Elective surgical repair
• Aortic rupture • Aortic dissection • Symptomatic aortic root dilation (may represent an impeding rupture)	• Aortic dilation >55 mm • Aortic dilation >50 mm in individuals with Marfan syndrome or bicuspid valves • Rate of growth >10 mm/year • Aortic insufficiency (decision largely based on diameter of aortic dilation)

Table 3.
Indications for emergent and elective surgical repair of aortic root dilation.

of growth of an aneurysm surpasses 10 mm/year, and if there is concurrent aortic insufficiency [1, 100]. In addition, patients who undergo aortic insufficiency repair who have concurrent aortic root dilation should be considered for aortic replacement at the time of their surgery—that is since 25% of patients with aortic root diameters >40 mm will eventually also require intervention for their aortic aneurysm [107].

4.2.2 Surgical interventions

As opposed to supravalvular aortic aneurysms, aortic root aneurysms involve the coronary ostia as well as the aortic valve, which have implications on the type of surgical procedure available for patients. There are two approaches for a surgical intervention: radical and conservative. In a radial surgical intervention the patient's aortic valve and root are replaced (commonly referred to as the Bentall procedure), whereas in conservative interventions only the aortic root is replaced [108].

The Bentall procedure involves replacing the aortic valve with a prosthetic valve, and thus has the caveat of requiring indefinite anticoagulation [5]. If patients have a high bleeding risk it may therefore be worthwhile investigating replacement of the aortic root while preserving the valve. In addition, it is important to note that a large number of patients with aortic root dilation are young (secondary to its association with Marfan syndrome), and therefore lifelong anticoagulation in cases such as these confers a cumulative bleeding risk. Preserving the aortic valve while surgically treating the aortic root dilatation is made possible by the development of two surgical procedures: the first is removing the aortic root while keeping the valve intact. The second method is through re-implantation of the aortic valve [5]. Both the Bentall procedure as well as aortic valve-preserving procedures have been shown to have comparable short and long-term outcomes with regards to the risk of death and valve associated complications. The main difference however is that patients undergoing valve sparing operations were significantly more likely to develop moderate to severe aortic regurgitation later [108].

In patients with both severe aortic stenosis and ascending aortic aneurysm, undergoing surgical aortic valve replacement (sAVR) and concomitant surgical intervention for aortic aneurysms above 4.5 cm is recommended by the American College of Cardiology (ACC) foundation guidelines [84]. However, in high-risk surgical patients, undergoing a transcatheter aortic valve replacement (TAVR) has become an alternative approach that obviates the need for parallel surgical aortic aneurysm intervention. This raises the concern for the safety of TAVR catheter-based delivery system in patients with aortic aneurysms since intraoperative rupture or dissection risk potentially increases. However, a clinical study showed that TAVR does not increase intraoperative aortic dissection/rupture risk or mortality with a median follow-up of 14 months [109]. Therefore, there are no recommendations against performing TAVR in patients with ascending aortic aneurysms.

Conflict of interest

None.

Author details

Ozan Unlu[1], Zaid I. Almarzooq[2], Diala Steitieh[1], Matthew Brandorff[1] and Parmanand Singh[3]*

1 Department of Medicine, Weill Cornell Medicine, New York, NY, USA

2 Department of Cardiology, Brigham and Women's Hospital, Boston, MA, USA

3 Department of Cardiology, Weill Cornell Medicine, New York, NY, USA

*Address all correspondence to: pas9062@med.cornell.edu

References

[1] Boyer JK, Gutierrez F, Braverman AC. Approach to the dilated aortic root. Current Opinion in Cardiology. 2004;**19**(6):563-569

[2] Roman MJ et al. Two-dimensional echocardiographic aortic root dimensions in normal children and adults. The American Journal of Cardiology. 1989;**64**(8):507-512

[3] Kim JB et al. Risk of aortic dissection in the moderately dilated ascending aorta. Journal of the American College of Cardiology. 2016;**68**(11):1209-1219

[4] Landenhed M et al. Risk profiles for aortic dissection and ruptured or surgically treated aneurysms: A prospective cohort study. Journal of the American Heart Association. 2015;**4**(1):e001513

[5] Nataf P, Lansac E. Dilation of the thoracic aorta: Medical and surgical management. Heart. 2006;**92**(9):1345-1352

[6] Douglas PS et al. ACCF/ASE/AHA/ASNC/HFSA/HRS/SCAI/SCCM/SCCT/SCMR 2011 Appropriate Use Criteria for Echocardiography. A report of the American College of Cardiology Foundation Appropriate Use Criteria Task Force, American Society of Echocardiography, American Heart Association, American Society of Nuclear Cardiology, Heart Failure Society of America, Heart Rhythm Society, Society for Cardiovascular Angiography and Interventions, Society of Critical Care Medicine, Society of Cardiovascular Computed Tomography, Society for Cardiovascular Magnetic Resonance American College of Chest Physicians. Journal of the American Society of Echocardiography. 2011;**24**(3):229-267

[7] Singh MN, Lacro RV. Recent clinical drug trials evidence in Marfan syndrome and clinical implications. The Canadian Journal of Cardiology. 2016;**32**(1):66-77

[8] Sakai LY et al. Purification and partial characterization of fibrillin, a cysteine-rich structural component of connective tissue microfibrils. The Journal of Biological Chemistry. 1991;**266**(22):14763-14770

[9] Judge DP, Dietz HC. Marfan's syndrome. Lancet. 2005;**366**(9501): 1965-1976

[10] Hilhorst-Hofstee Y et al. The clinical spectrum of missense mutations of the first aspartic acid of cbEGF-like domains in fibrillin-1 including a recessive family. Human Mutation. 2010;**31**(12):E1915-E1927

[11] Dietz H. Marfan syndrome. 2001. In: Adam MP, Ardinger HH, Pagon RA, et al., editors. GeneReviews® [Internet]. Seattle, WA: University of Washington, Seattle; 1993-2018. Available from: https://www.ncbi.nlm.nih.gov/books/NBK1335/

[12] Pyeritz RE. Recent progress in understanding the natural and clinical histories of the Marfan syndrome. Trends in Cardiovascular Medicine. 2016;**26**(5):423-428

[13] Akhurst RJ. TGF beta signaling in health and disease. Nature Genetics. 2004;**36**(8):790-792

[14] Loeys BL et al. A syndrome of altered cardiovascular, craniofacial, neurocognitive and skeletal development caused by mutations in TGFBR1 or TGFBR2. Nature Genetics. 2005;**37**(3):275-281

[15] Mizuguchi T et al. Heterozygous TGFBR2 mutations in Marfan syndrome. Nature Genetics. 2004;**36**(8):855-860

[16] De Paepe A et al. Revised diagnostic criteria for the Marfan syndrome. American Journal of Medical Genetics. 1996;**62**(4):417-426

[17] Loeys BL et al. The revised Ghent nosology for the Marfan syndrome. Journal of Medical Genetics. 2010;**47**(7):476-485

[18] Roman MJ et al. Prognostic significance of the pattern of aortic root dilation in the Marfan syndrome. Journal of the American College of Cardiology. 1993;**22**(5):1470-1476

[19] Roberts WC. The congenitally bicuspid aortic valve. A study of 85 autopsy cases. The American Journal of Cardiology. 1970;**26**(1):72-83

[20] Cripe L et al. Bicuspid aortic valve is heritable. Journal of the American College of Cardiology. 2004;**44**(1):138-143

[21] Warnes CA et al. ACC/AHA 2008 guidelines for the management of adults with congenital heart disease: A report of the American College of Cardiology/ American Heart Association Task Force on Practice Guidelines (Writing Committee to Develop Guidelines on the Management of Adults with Congenital Heart Disease). Developed in collaboration with the American Society of Echocardiography, Heart Rhythm Society, International Society for Adult Congenital Heart Disease, Society for Cardiovascular Angiography and Interventions, and Society of Thoracic Surgeons. Journal of the American College of Cardiology. 2008;**52**(23):e143-e263

[22] Ayad RF et al. Accuracy of two-dimensional echocardiography in determining aortic valve structure in patients >50 years of age having aortic valve replacement for aortic stenosis. The American Journal of Cardiology. 2011;**108**(11):1589-1599

[23] Nishimura RA et al. 2014 AHA/ ACC guideline for the management of patients with valvular heart disease: Executive summary: A report of the American College of Cardiology/ American Heart Association Task Force on Practice Guidelines. Circulation. 2014;**129**(23):2440-2492

[24] Verma S, Siu SC. Aortic dilatation in patients with bicuspid aortic valve. The New England Journal of Medicine. 2014;**370**(20):1920-1929

[25] Bonderman D et al. Mechanisms underlying aortic dilatation in congenital aortic valve malformation. Circulation. 1999;**99**(16):2138-2143

[26] Ward C. Clinical significance of the bicuspid aortic valve. Heart. 2000;**83**(1):81-85

[27] MacCarrick G et al. Loeys-Dietz syndrome: A primer for diagnosis and management. Genetics in Medicine. 2014;**16**(8):576-587

[28] Meester JAN et al. Differences in manifestations of Marfan syndrome, Ehlers-Danlos syndrome, and Loeys-Dietz syndrome. Annals of cardiothoracic surgery. 2017;**6**(6):582-594

[29] Attias D et al. Comparison of clinical presentations and outcomes between patients with TGFBR2 and FBN1 mutations in Marfan syndrome and related disorders. Circulation. 2009;**120**(25):2541-2549

[30] Erbel R et al. 2014 ESC guidelines on the diagnosis and treatment of aortic diseases: Document covering acute and chronic aortic diseases of the thoracic and abdominal aorta of the adult. The Task Force for the Diagnosis and Treatment of Aortic Diseases of the European Society of Cardiology (ESC). European Heart Journal. 2014;**35**(41):2873-2926

[31] Beighton P et al. Ehlers-Danlos syndromes: Revised nosology,

Villefranche, 1997. Ehlers-Danlos National Foundation (USA) and Ehlers-Danlos Support Group (UK). American Journal of Medical Genetics. 1998;**77**(1):31-37

[32] Freeman LA et al. CT and MRI assessment of the aortic root and ascending aorta. AJR. American Journal of Roentgenology. 2013;**200**(6):W581-W592

[33] Hiratzka LF et al. 2010 ACCF/AHA/AATS/ACR/ASA/SCA/SCAI/SIR/STS/SVM guidelines for the diagnosis and management of patients with thoracic aortic disease. A report of the American College of Cardiology Foundation/American Heart Association Task Force on Practice Guidelines, American Association for Thoracic Surgery, American College of Radiology, American Stroke Association, Society of Cardiovascular Anesthesiologists, Society for Cardiovascular Angiography and Interventions, Society of Interventional Radiology, Society of Thoracic Surgeons, and Society for Vascular Medicine. Journal of the American College of Cardiology. 2010;**55**(14):e27-e129

[34] Henry WL, Gardin JM, Ware JH. Echocardiographic measurements in normal subjects from infancy to old age. Circulation. 1980;**62**(5):1054-1061

[35] Rozendaal L et al. Marfan syndrome in children and adolescents: An adjusted nomogram for screening aortic root dilatation. Heart. 1998;**79**(1):69-72

[36] Sawabe M et al. Age is a major pathobiological determinant of aortic dilatation: A large autopsy study of community deaths. Journal of Atherosclerosis and Thrombosis. 2011;**18**(2):157-165

[37] Okamoto RJ et al. The influence of mechanical properties on wall stress and distensibility of the dilated ascending aorta. The Journal of Thoracic and Cardiovascular Surgery. 2003;**126**(3):842-850

[38] O'Rourke MF, Hashimoto J. Mechanical factors in arterial aging: A clinical perspective. Journal of the American College of Cardiology. 2007;**50**(1):1-13

[39] Wang M et al. Proinflammatory profile within the grossly normal aged human aortic wall. Hypertension. 2007;**50**(1):219-227

[40] Vasan RS, Larson MG, Levy D. Determinants of echocardiographic aortic root size. The Framingham Heart Study. Circulation. 1995;**91**(3):734-740

[41] Covella M et al. Echocardiographic aortic root dilatation in hypertensive patients: A systematic review and meta-analysis. Journal of Hypertension. 2014;**32**(10):1928-1935; discussion 1935

[42] Iskandar A, Thompson PD. A meta-analysis of aortic root size in elite athletes. Circulation. 2013;**127**(7):791-798

[43] Mitchell GF et al. Aortic diameter, wall stiffness, and wave reflection in systolic hypertension. Hypertension. 2008;**51**(1):105-111

[44] Ingelsson E et al. Aortic root diameter and longitudinal blood pressure tracking. Hypertension. 2008;**52**(3):473-477

[45] Lam CS et al. Aortic root remodeling over the adult life course: Longitudinal data from the Framingham Heart Study. Circulation. 2010;**122**(9):884-890

[46] Gornik HL, Creager MA. Aortitis. Circulation. 2008;**117**(23):3039-3051

[47] Aminov RI. A brief history of the antibiotic era: Lessons learned and challenges for the future. Frontiers in Microbiology. 2010;**1**:134

[48] Soravia-Dunand VA, Loo VG, Salit IE. Aortitis due to *Salmonella*: Report of 10 cases and comprehensive review of the literature. Clinical Infectious Diseases. 1999;**29**(4):862-868

[49] Feigl D, Feigl A, Edwards JE. Mycotic aneurysms of the aortic root. A pathologic study of 20 cases. Chest. 1986;**90**(4):553-557

[50] Restrepo CS et al. Aortitis: Imaging spectrum of the infectious and inflammatory conditions of the aorta. Radiographics. 2011;**31**(2):435-451

[51] Paulo N, Cascarejo J, Vouga L. Syphilitic aneurysm of the ascending aorta. Interactive Cardiovascular and Thoracic Surgery. 2012; **14**(2):223-225

[52] Heggtveit HA. Syphilitic aortitis. A clinicopathologic autopsy study of 100 cases, 1950 to 1960. Circulation. 1964;**29**:346-355

[53] Glaziou P et al. Global epidemiology of tuberculosis. Seminars in Respiratory and Critical Care Medicine. 2013;**34**(1):3-16

[54] Sharma D et al. Dissecting aortic root aneurysm and severe aortic regurgitation following pulmonary tuberculosis. Egyptian Journal of Chest Diseases and Tuberculosis. 2014;**63**(2):523-527

[55] Javed MA, Sheppard MN, Pepper J. Aortic root dilation secondary to giant cell aortitis in a human immunodeficiency virus-positive patient. European Journal of Cardio-Thoracic Surgery. 2006;**30**(2):400-401

[56] Haenen F, Laga S, Rodrigus I. Q fever infection: Inflammatory aortic root aneurysm in an HIV positive patient. Acta Cardiologica. 2012;**67**(2):261-264

[57] Ozkan Y. Cardiac involvement in ankylosing spondylitis. Journal of Clinical Medical Research. 2016;**8**(6):427-430

[58] Roldan CA et al. Aortic root disease and valve disease associated with ankylosing spondylitis. Journal of the American College of Cardiology. 1998;**32**(5):1397-1404

[59] Sharma A et al. Relapsing polychondritis: A review. Clinical Rheumatology. 2013;**32**(11):1575-1583

[60] Selim AG et al. Active aortitis in relapsing polychondritis. Journal of Clinical Pathology. 2001;**54**(11):890-892

[61] Sharma A et al. Successful treatment of aortic root dilatation in a patient with relapsing polychondritis. Clinical Rheumatology. 2013;**32**(Suppl 1):S59-S61

[62] Mason JC. Takayasu arteritis—Advances in diagnosis and management. Nature Reviews Rheumatology. 2010;**6**(7):406-415

[63] Murayama M et al. A case of severe aortic regurgitation caused by Takayasu's arteritis showing end-diastolic opening of aortic valve. CASE. 2018;**2**(6):248-253

[64] Kaku Y et al. Surgery for aortic regurgitation and aortic root dilatation in Takayasu arteritis. Asian Cardiovascular & Thoracic Annals. 2015;**23**(8):901-906

[65] Iarussi D et al. Association of left ventricular hypertrophy and aortic dilation in patients with acute thoracic aortic dissection. Angiology. 2001;**52**(7):447-455

[66] Cuspidi C et al. Clinical and prognostic value of hypertensive cardiac damage in the PAMELA study. Hypertension Research. 2017;**40**(4):329-335

[67] Davies RR et al. Yearly rupture or dissection rates for thoracic aortic

aneurysms: Simple prediction based on size. The Annals of Thoracic Surgery. 2002;**73**(1):17-27; discussion 27-28

[68] Liddicoat JE et al. Ascending aortic aneurysms. Review of 100 consecutive cases. Circulation. 1975;**52**(2 Suppl): I202-I209

[69] Erbel R, Eggebrecht H. Aortic dimensions and the risk of dissection. Heart. 2006;**92**(1):137-142

[70] Najafi H et al. Aortic insufficiency secondary to aortic root aneurysm or dissection. Archives of Surgery. 1975;**110**(11):1401-1407

[71] Pabisiak K et al. Ascending aorta aneurysm as a cause of superior vena cava syndrome. Polski Merkuriusz Lekarski. 2014;**37**(218):104-107

[72] Eccles SR, Banks J, Kumar P. Ascending aortic aneurysm causing hoarse voice: A variant of Ortner's syndrome. BML Case Reports. 2012;**2012**:bcr2012007111

[73] Kim JH et al. A patient with dysphagia due to an aortic aneurysm. Korean Circulation Journal. 2009;**39**(6):258-260

[74] Kumar A et al. Vascular airway compression management in a case of aortic arch and descending thoracic aortic aneurysm. Annals of Cardiac Anaesthesia. 2016;**19**(3):568-571

[75] Hahn RT et al. Association of aortic dilation with regurgitant, stenotic and functionally normal bicuspid aortic valves. Journal of the American College of Cardiology. 1992;**19**(2):283-288

[76] Pretre R, Von Segesser LK. Aortic dissection. Lancet. 1997;**349**(9063):1461-1464

[77] Hagan PG et al. The International Registry of Acute Aortic Dissection (IRAD): New insights into an old disease. JAMA. 2000;**283**(7):897-903

[78] Mehta RH et al. Acute type A aortic dissection in the elderly: Clinical characteristics, management, and outcomes in the current era. Journal of the American College of Cardiology. 2002;**40**(4):685-692

[79] Rogers AM et al. Sensitivity of the aortic dissection detection risk score, a novel guideline-based tool for identification of acute aortic dissection at initial presentation: Results from the international registry of acute aortic dissection. Circulation. 2011;**123**(20):2213-2218

[80] Sun D, Mehta S. Hemoptysis caused by erosion of thoracic aortic aneurysm. CMAJ. 2010;**182**(4):E186

[81] Gerrard AD, Batool S, Isaacs P. Ruptured thoracic aneurysm causing hematemesis. ACG Case Reports Journal. 2016;**3**(4):e182

[82] Fukui T et al. Cardiac tamponade secondary to rupture of a distal aortic arch aneurysm. The Japanese Journal of Thoracic and Cardiovascular Surgery. 2002;**50**(5):227-230

[83] Roman MJ et al. Aortic root dilatation as a cause of isolated, severe aortic regurgitation. Prevalence, clinical and echocardiographic patterns, and relation to left ventricular hypertrophy and function. Annals of Internal Medicine. 1987;**106**(6):800-807

[84] Hiratzka LF et al. ACCF/AHA/AATS/ACR/ASA/SCA/SCAI/SIR/STS/SVM guidelines for the diagnosis and management of patients with thoracic aortic disease: A report of the American College of Cardiology Foundation/American Heart Association Task Force on Practice Guidelines, American Association for Thoracic Surgery, American College of Radiology,

American Stroke Association, Society of Cardiovascular Anesthesiologists, Society for Cardiovascular Angiography and Interventions, Society of Interventional Radiology, Society of Thoracic Surgeons, and Society for Vascular Medicine. Circulation. 2010, 2010;**121**(13):e266-e369

[85] Saliba E, Sia Y. The ascending aortic aneurysm: When to intervene? International Journal of Cardiology. Heart & Vasculature. 2015;**6**:91-100. DOI: 10.1016/j.ijcha.2015.01.009. eCollection 2015 Mar 1

[86] Vasan RS et al. Echocardiographic reference values for aortic root size: The Framingham Heart Study. Journal of the American Society of Echocardiography. 1995;**8**(6):793-800

[87] Goldstein SA et al. Multimodality imaging of diseases of the thoracic aorta in adults: From the American Society of Echocardiography and the European Association of Cardiovascular Imaging: Endorsed by the Society of Cardiovascular Computed Tomography and Society for Cardiovascular Magnetic Resonance. Journal of the American Society of Echocardiography. 2015;**28**(2):119-182

[88] Solomon SD, Wu J, Gillam LD. Essential Echocardiography: A Companion to Braunwald's Heart Disease. Philadelphia, PA: Elsevier Health Sciences; 2017

[89] Steinberg CR, Archer M, Steinberg I. Measurement of the abdominal aorta after intravenous aortography in health and arteriosclerotic peripheral vascular disease. The American Journal of Roentgenology, Radium Therapy, and Nuclear Medicine. 1965; **95**(3):703-708

[90] Nayak KS et al. Spiral balanced steady-state free precession cardiac imaging. Magnetic Resonance in Medicine. 2005;**53**(6):1468-1473

[91] Carr JC et al. Cine MR angiography of the heart with segmented true fast imaging with steady-state precession. Radiology. 2001;**219**(3):828-834

[92] Gebker R et al. Comparison of different MRI techniques for the assessment of thoracic aortic pathology: 3D contrast enhanced MR angiography, turbo spin echo and balanced steady state free precession. The International Journal of Cardiovascular Imaging. 2007;**23**(6):747-756

[93] Burman ED, Keegan J, Kilner PJ. Aortic root measurement by cardiovascular magnetic resonance: Specification of planes and lines of measurement and corresponding normal values. Circulation. Cardiovascular Imaging. 2008;**1**(2):104-113

[94] Brenner DJ, Hall EJ. Computed tomography—An increasing source of radiation exposure. The New England Journal of Medicine. 2007;**357**(22):2277-2284

[95] Di Cesare E et al. CT and MR imaging of the thoracic aorta. Open medicine (Warsaw, Poland). 2016;**11**(1):143-151

[96] Litmanovich D et al. CT and MRI in diseases of the aorta. AJR - American Journal of Roentgenology. 2009;**193**(4):928-940

[97] Hanneman K et al. Pre- and post-operative imaging of the aortic root. Radiographics. 2016;**36**(1):19-37

[98] McLarty AJ, Bishawi M, Yelika SB, Shroyer AL, Romeiser J. Surveillance of moderate-size aneurysms of the thoracic aorta. Journal of Cardiothoracic Surgery. 2015;**10**:17

[99] Sodickson A. Recurrent CT, cumulative radiation exposure, and associated radiation-induced cancer risks from CT of adults. Radiology. 2009;**251**(1):175-184

[100] Elefteriades JA. Natural history of thoracic aortic aneurysms: Indications for surgery, and surgical versus nonsurgical risks. The Annals of Thoracic Surgery. 2002;**74**(5):S1877-S1880; discussion S1892-S1898

[101] Jondeau G et al. Marfan syndrome. Archives des Maladies du Coeur et des Vaisseaux. 2003;**96**(11):1081-1088

[102] Danyi P, Elefteriades JA, Jovin IS. Medical therapy of thoracic aortic aneurysms: Are we there yet? Circulation. 2011;**124**(13):1469-1476

[103] Rossi-Foulkes R et al. Phenotypic features and impact of beta blocker or calcium antagonist therapy on aortic lumen size in the Marfan syndrome. The American Journal of Cardiology. 1999;**83**(9):1364-1368

[104] Aronow WS. Treatment of thoracic aortic aneurysm. Annals of Translational Medicine. 2018;**6**(3):66

[105] Stone NJ et al. 2013 ACC/AHA guideline on the treatment of blood cholesterol to reduce atherosclerotic cardiovascular risk in adults: A report of the American College of Cardiology/American Heart Association Task Force on Practice Guidelines. Journal of the American College of Cardiology. 2014;**63**(25 Pt B):2889-2934

[106] Mitchell JH et al. Task force 8: Classification of sports. Journal of the American College of Cardiology. 2005;**45**(8):1364-1367

[107] Isselbacher EM. Thoracic and abdominal aortic aneurysms. Circulation. 2005;**111**(6):816-828

[108] Lim JY et al. Surgical management of aortic root dilatation with advanced aortic regurgitation: Bentall operation versus valve-sparing procedure. The Korean Journal of Thoracic and Cardiovascular Surgery. 2012;**45**(3):141-147

[109] Rylski B et al. Transcatheter aortic valve implantation in patients with ascending aortic dilatation: Safety of the procedure and mid-term follow-up. European Journal of Cardio-Thoracic Surgery. 2014;**46**(2):228-233

Chapter 2

Challenges for Intelligent Data Analysis Methods in Medical Image Analysis during Surgical Interventions of Aneurysms

Abdullah Al Amoudi, Shankar Srinivasan and Mohamed Yacin Sikkandar

Abstract

Aortic aneurysms (AA) can be the primary cause of over 10,000 deaths and indirect cause for another 18,000 deaths annually in the USA as per the recent data released by the Centers for Disease Control and Prevention. Among the several factors related to high mortality, imaging methods and intervention procedures could be important. The commonly used diagnostic imaging methods of aneurysms are computed tomography (CT), magnet resonance imaging (MRI), ultrasound (US), digital subtraction angiography (DSA) and amalgamation of fluoro-D-glucose (FDG) integrated with positron emission tomography (PET) and/or CT and PET with CT or MRI. Several research findings indicate that diagnostic efficiency of different imaging methods differ. As intervention procedures depend upon diagnosis, the choice of appropriate diagnostic imaging method for a given case is very important. If the critical characteristics of the swelling are not detected due to the choice of unsuitable imaging method, interventions may not be very suitable. The American College of Radiologists (ACR) prescribed some appropriateness guidelines for diagnostic imaging. Not complying with them fully or partially may also be a mortality factor. This chapter is written with recent research findings in the field of intelligent data analysis for medical applications supported by case studies and practical examples.

Keywords: diagnosis, aneurysm, imaging modality, guidelines, mortality

1. Introduction

Aneurysm was the primary cause of more than 10,597 deaths and a contributing cause of over 17,215 deaths in the USA in 2009 [1], shown in **Figure 1**. Some essential details on aneurysm, its diagnosis, factors of influence and prevention and treatment are described by Nordqvist [2]. The author gives a more detailed description of aneurysm. The disease occurs when an artery or cardiac chamber swells. This results in the damage of artery or weakness of its walls. The swelling balloons out at its weakest point resulting from increasing blood pressure. This means there should be a threshold pressure above which only ballooning out

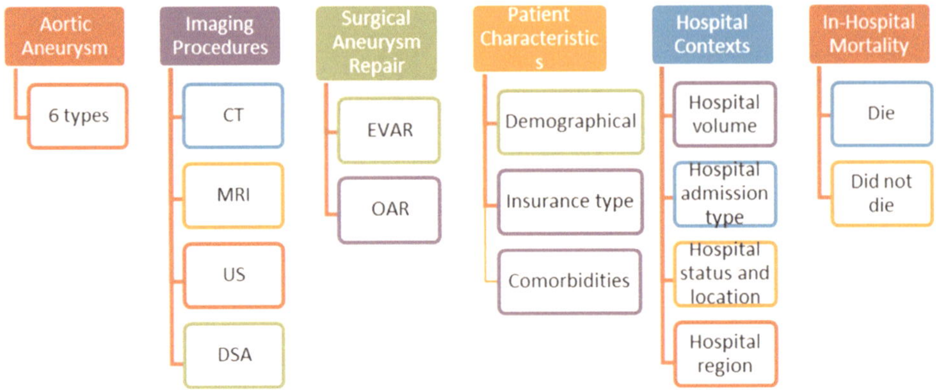

Figure 1.
Subcategorization of data elements used in this study.

happens. Although small swellings may be confined to a small area of the artery, large ones can extend along the whole length of the affected area. The balloon may become too large, and it may rupture when pressure build-up continues. Furthermore, a threshold point is indicated for the rupture. The rupture naturally leads to hemorrhage and other complications and even sudden death. Although aneurysm can occur in any part of the body, it is more common in the arteries, particularly in the aorta. True aneurysms can be atherosclerotic, syphilitic, congenital or ventricular following transmural myocardial infarctions and can occur in any of the three walls of the artery.

False aneurysm (pseudo-aneurysm) is also possible when there is complete leaking of blood out of an artery or vein confined to the tissue surrounding the vessel. Eventually, this blood-filled cavity may clot to seal the leak, or it may rupture out of the surrounding tissue. Trauma can be caused by punctures in the artery created by knife, bullet and so forth. Pseudo-aneurysms can be caused by percutaneous surgical procedures like coronary angiography or arterial grafting or an injection into the artery. Aneurysms are classified according to their morphology or by location. Morphologically, saccular aneurysms are spherical, 5–20 cm in diameter, partially or fully filled by thrombus and involve only a portion of the vessel wall. Fusiform types are spindle-shaped, with varying diameter up to 20 cm and with varying length, involving large portions of ascending and transverse aortic arch, abdominal aorta or iliac arteries.

Aneurysms, by location, could be arterial or venous, the former being more common. Aneurysms related to heart can be coronary artery aneurysms, ventricular aneurysms and aneurysms of sinus of Valsalva. Aneurysms following cardiac surgery also occur. Related to aorta, abdominal aortic aneurysm and thoracic aortic aneurysm can occur. Results of some studies show that about 25% of aneurysms occur in the thoracic area [3]. Related to the brain, cerebral, berry or Charcot-Bouchard aneurysms can occur. Cerebral aneurysm (intracranial or brain aneurysm) is more common at the base of the brain and more common in the anterior cerebral artery, especially in the internal carotid artery. Aneurysms can occur in the legs, especially in popliteal arteries. In the kidney, renal artery or intra-parenchymal aneurysms can occur. However, renal and leg aneurysms are rare. A comprehensive list of various types of aneurysms is given in **Table 1**.

Some studies show that mortalities vary with patient characteristics as well as the specific hospital contexts. Patient characteristics, such as gender, age, and comorbidities of some aortic aneurysm types, have been studied. Hospital contexts

Affected region	Aneurysm nomenclature
Aortic aneurysm	Thoracic aortic aneurysm Ruptured thoracic aortic aneurysm Thoracicoabdominal aortic aneurysm Ruptured thoracicoabdominal aortic aneurysm Abdominal aortic aneurysm Ruptured abdominal aortic aneurysm
Cranial and neck aneurysm artery	Cerebral artery aneurysm Ruptured cerebral artery aneurysm Ruptured syphilitic cerebral aneurysm Congenital cerebral artery aneurysm Carotid artery aneurysm Subclavian artery aneurysm
Intrathoracic aneurysm arteries	Heart aneurysm Coronary artery aneurysm Pulmonary artery aneurysm Mediastinal and spinal artery aneurysm
Intra-abdominal and pelvic aneurysm arteries	Renal artery aneurysm Splenic artery aneurysm Visceral artery aneurysm Iliac artery aneurysm
Upper extremity arteries	Brachial artery aneurysm Radial artery aneurysm
Lower extremity arteries	Femoral artery Popliteal artery

Table 1.
Comprehensive list of aneurysm types.

include type, location, educational qualifications and experience of health-care professionals and patient volume. However, not many studies have reported on the influence of using various types of imaging modalities and their capability to lead and guide aneurysm repair procedures to decrease the mortality rate of aortic aneurysm patients. One of the important aspects in hospital context is its adherence with the American College of Radiologists (ACR) guideline especially on medical imaging methods and patients safety aspects. The lack of protocols and costs have been cited as important reasons for not practising the most desirable or appropriate imaging methods in the case of aneurysm [4]. Obviously this affects the extent of compliance with ACR. However, not many studies have been reported on the influence of extent of compliance of medical imaging guidelines of ACR on the in-hospital mortality of aortic aneurysm patients.

Scientific knowledge is the basis of diagnostic and treatment procedures. It determines the diagnostic methods to be used for accurate assessment of the disease so that effective treatment procedure can be determined.

Imaging is a scientific method used for the diagnosis of aneurysm. If appropriate imaging methods are not used, the treatment outcome may be negative. The guidelines of ACR are relevant in this respect. Hospitals are rated according to their compliance with ACR, and its influence on in-hospital mortality is evaluated. The relationship between in-patient hospital mortality and aneurysm and the relationship between compliance with ACR and in-hospital mortality of aneurysm patients point to the importance of evidence-based diagnosis and treatment procedure. Thus, effectiveness of diagnosis using imaging techniques and its outcome in terms of mortality for hospitalized patients forms the most important components of the findings.

Patient safety is an important aspect of both diagnosis and treatment. Radiation exposure in terms of type, dose and duration and conditions under which imaging is done are of critical importance, and ACR has critical points on these aspects. This applies to treatment also. So, ACR compliance level and other hospital contexts determine the extent to which patient safety is cared for. This is an aspect derivable from the findings of this work. Thus, some of the six dimensions of heath-care quality are evaluated in this work.

So, the following questions are relevant:

1. How do the algorithms of these imaging methods determine the efficiency and effectiveness of diagnosis in the case of aneurysm?

2. Why is DSA preferred over other imaging methods for the diagnosis of aneurysm?

3. Is there any risk of higher mortality or reduction in mortality by not following/following ACR appropriateness guidelines for diagnostic imaging?

This chapter tries to answer the above questions based on our recent research findings.

2. Efficiency and effectiveness of diagnosis of imaging methods

Commonly used diagnostic imaging methods of aneurysms are computed tomography (CT), magnetic resonance imaging (MRI), ultrasound (US), digital subtraction angiography (DSA) and combinations of FDG with PET and/or CT and PET with CT or MRI. Many research findings indicate that diagnostic efficiency of different imaging methods differs. As intervention procedures depend upon diagnosis, the choice of appropriate diagnostic imaging method for a given case is very important. If the critical characteristics of the swelling are not detected due to the choice of unsuitable imaging method, interventions may not be very suitable. In this study, six types of aortic aneurysms are covered. These are ruptured and intact thoracic aortic aneurysms (rTA and TA), ruptured and intact abdominal aortic aneurysms (rAAA and AAA) and ruptured and intact thoracicoabdominal aortic aneurysms (rTAA and TAA). Surgical repairs by OAR and EVAR are the intervention procedures. The main imaging procedures are CT, MRI, ultrasound and DSA. The subcategorization of data elements is given in **Figure 1**.

Recent advances have made computed tomography angiography (CTA) and magnetic resonance angiography (MRA) as the most useful diagnostic tools for aortic aneurysm. These developments have helped to reduce the procedural risks of transarterial catheterization. Cross-sectional images provide information on the affected blood vessel and length of its affected part, total aortic diameter and diameter of the artery, true vascular diameter which includes patent lumen, the extent of formation of mural thrombus, the distance of diseased wall from critical aortic branches and extravascular pathology. This imaging method is used as a single procedure for diagnosis, procedure planning and post-operative monitoring. It has helped to reduce the rate of morbidity and mortality. Catheter-based angiography is used as an adjunct to treatment procedures. Integrated with contemporary cross-sectional imaging, this method includes uses of carbon dioxide angiography and intravascular ultrasound methods. Multiple imaging is done in which one pre-contrast imaging series and at least one contrast-enhanced imaging are included. Although contrast injection protocols include a number of parameters, the critical challenge is the optimal delivery of appropriate quantity of contrast to the volume of interest. These protocols need to be carefully determined for each specific situation. CTA has a definite edge over MRA in many respects. Renal impairment prevents the use of iodine contrast agents. Renal protective strategies are used for its mitigation, with a doubtful benefit at times.

CTA is a quick, reliable, simple and non-invasive diagnostic tool for aneurysms and can effectively replace conventional angiography [3]. Therefore, according to Prestigiacomo et al., 3-D CTA can be used as an initial screening tool in place of DSA. Sensitivity and predictive values of 100% were obtained by them. Sensitivity of 2D and 3D CTA to detect very small aneurysms was 98–100% compared to 95% for DSA [5]. CTA accuracy was also 99–100%. Based on these findings, Villablanca et al. recommended the use of CTA with commercial detectors to detect very small aneurysms [6]. Even without pre-operative angiography, pre-operative 3D CTA (instead of DSA angiography) can provide good anatomical information for microsurgical interventions of aneurysms, as was concluded by González-Darder et al. [7]. Forsting in 2005 concluded that CTA can effectively replace DSA and even MRA for diagnosis aneurysm [8]. Hoh et al. demonstrated the possibility of using only CTA instead of DSA for diagnosis and pretreatment planning in patients with ruptured and unruptured aneurysms in Massachusetts General Hospital [9]. In the findings of Karamessini et al., CTA had sensitivity, specificity, positive predictive, negative predictive and accuracy values of 88.7, 100, 100, 80.7, and 92.3%, respectively. The corresponding values for DSA were 87.8, 98, 97.7, 89.1, and 92.9%, respectively [10]. Based on these findings, the authors concluded that CTA and DSA were equally good for detection of aneurysms of 3 mm or more. With 100% detection accuracy, CTA is also useful to detect AcoA and MCA bifurcation aneurysms. According to Matsumoto et al., 3D CTA can effectively replace conventional catheter angiography in the diagnosis and surgery of most ruptured aneurysms [11]. Furthermore, a recent systematic review done by our group in 2015 also supports the use of CTA as an effective substitute for other imaging methods, at least to some extent, in the treatment and diagnosis of AAA [12]. In measuring the volume of aneurysms, CTA, MRA and rotational DSA produced statistically non-significant differences and hence can be considered equally as per the report of Piotin et al. [13].

On the other hand, in a comparative study, Biasi et al. found CTA inadequate to detect small aneurysms occasionally and therefore recommended DSA/3D rotational angiography [14]. Stavropoulos et al. also considered CTA inferior in detecting small aneurysms, and the use of DSA should be continued. Difficulty of detecting small aneurysms using CTA has been reported by many other workers [15]. According to latest study in 2015 by Chung et al., multi-slice 3D CTA offers better image resolution and is hence more useful than single-slice CTA to detect aortic aneurysms for post-EVAR [16]. In another finding, van Gelder [17] supported further investigation of small aneurysms detected by CTA if there is no pretest probability of ruptured aneurysm. Very low probability of clinically significant aneurysms can be detected by CTA when screening is done for unruptured aneurysms.

Some technological improvements include Sailer et al. in 2014 on using fluoroscopy image fusion guidance for CTA in endovascular interventions to reduce iodine contrast dose and procedure duration [18], Deák et al. on automated systems for detection of aortic aneurysms in CTA images [19] and Wada et al. 2014 on combining 3D CTA with 2D CT imaging guidance for clipping surgery [20].

2.1 Why is DSA preferred over other imaging methods for aneurysm detection?

Many research works and reports [21–24] indicate distinct preference for DSA over other imaging methods when diagnosing a variety of aneurysms. Specific reasons may be related to the availability of instruments, specifically trained staff, costs, convenience, etc. In the case of some specific types of aneurysms, DSA has been shown to be the most suitable one for maximum efficiency and effectiveness. These factors are discussed using scientific evidence.

High resolution makes conventional angiography the most desirable diagnostic tool for aortic aneurysm. It is done at the earliest opportunity of patient presentation after bleeding. With haemorrhage risk being high within the first 24 hours, an early angiogram is necessary for therapeutic decisions. Aortic angiography can locate lesions, reveal the size and shape of aneurysm, detect presence of multiple aneurysms, examine vascular anatomy and its collaterals and evaluate the presence of vasospasm and its intensity.

Comparisons of CTA and DSA done by many workers have been discussed above. Other works related to DSA are reviewed here. More often, DSA is used as a confirmatory or extended test of other imaging methods. For example, although 3D CTA compared very well with DSA, in the experiment, DSA was used for confirmation of the results obtained with 3D CTA in the work of Thurnher et al. [25]. The 3D rotational reconstructed DSA images can improve the assessment of aneurysms [26]. Although CTA can add value to DSA, it can never replace it [27]. In one finding by van Rooij et al., 3D rotational angiography (3DRA) was found superior to DSA, and hence they suggested it as the new gold standard [28]. However, according to Zhang et al. contrast-enhanced dual-energy CTA had better diagnostic image quality at lower radiation dose than 3D DSA. Based on their research [29], Defillo et al. concluded that indocyanine green video-angiography (ICGV) had distinct advantages over intraoperative catheter DSA with respect to rapid feedback and visualizing of local perforators [30]. DSA had better visualization of residual aneurysm and parent artery stenosis which did not limit flow. Based on these findings, they recommended the combined use of the two imaging tools. On the other hand, due to the absence of small neck remnants and some residual aneurysms by ICGV, DSA is necessary for quality of surgery assessment in complex aneurysms. Better image quality is possible with lower dose of radiation, according to the results obtained by Pearl et al. [31].

CO2-DSA gave better results than conventional DS in detecting Type I and Type II direct endoleaks in EVAR procedure. This is because CO2-DSA had higher sensitivity and specificity than conventional DSA [32]. In the studies of Wacker et al., in 2014, C-arm CT is used as a supplementary imaging tool with DSA for better localization and classification of endoleaks than DSA alone in EVAR repair [33].

When EVAR was done using single imaging methods, DSA was most preferred followed by US, CT, and MRI in the decreasing order. When two imaging methods were combined, DSA with US recorded the highest imaging frequency. This was followed by DSA + CT and DSA + MRI. The same trend was observed in the case of OAR also. OAR combinations recorded higher frequencies than EVAR combinations, as OAR was the preferred intervention procedure.

The trend was maintained for each aneurysm type as well. In **Table 2**, overall frequency was highest for AAA followed by TA, rAAA, and TAA in the decreasing order. This reflects the relative incidence and prevalence of aneurysm type rather than any preference of imaging for a specific aneurysm type. More than 70% of all imaging and interventions were done on AAA followed by about 21% for TAA, together accounting for about 90% of all aneurysm care.

Medical imaging modalities associated with interventional repair	Frequency	Valid percent	Cumulative percent
	n	%	%
EVAR + CT	38	0.1	0.1
EVAR + MRI	6	0.0	0.1
EVAR + US	259	0.7	0.8
EVAR + DSA	7718	20.2	21.0
EVAR + DSA + CT	95	0.2	21.2
EVAR + DSA + MRI	6	0.0	21.2
EVAR + DSA + US	676	1.8	23.0
OAR + CT	485	1.3	24.3
OAR + MRI	106	0.3	24.5
OAR + US	4620	12.1	36.6
OAR + DSA	20,865	54.5	91.1
OAR + DSA + CT	292	0.8	91.9
OAR + DSA + MRI	69	0.2	92.1
OAR + DSA + US	3028	7.9	100.0
Total	38,263	100.0	

Table 2.
Imaging frequencies for different aortic aneurysm types.

2.2 Is there a higher mortality risk if ACR appropriateness guidelines for diagnostic imaging are not complied with? Alternatively, can it be shown that compliance with ACR guidelines reduced mortality risks?

In Canada, ultrasound screening of 65–75-year-old men is done and is cost-effective. Relative risk of AAA-related mortality is 0.49 for this group compared to no screen. There is little benefit by screening of men beyond 75 years old. Screening of women over 75 years is not recommended. Individualized check-up of women over 65 years is adequate. No follow-up screening is required for AAA size less than 3 cm. Although annual screening of individuals with 3–4.4 cm is routinely done, evidence for this is weak. Screening every 2 years may be enough. Screening for popliteal aneurysm may be beneficial. There is no benefit by screening men or women less than 65 years. Physical examination can supplement screening wherever necessary. As advances in surgery techniques reduce AAA-related mortality rates, the cost-effectiveness of screening needs to be reviewed periodically.

A set of guidelines on clinical practices for endovascular AAA repair was given by Walker et al. [34]. The guidelines deal with endovascular repair, its indications and contradictions, EVAR requirements of patients, procedural assessment before repair containing detailed imaging methods and scoring systems, endograft types and their suitability, technical aspects of surgical procedure and post-operative management. Another set of guidelines on the same topic was published for European Society for Vascular Surgery [35]. There was also an earlier set of guidelines of Society for Vascular Nursing (SVN) Task Force published by Smith et al. [36]. This covers mostly the nursing and patient care aspects of pre-operative, intraoperative and post-operative stages. The guidelines use evidence-based best practice approach. A set of guidelines for peripheral arterial disease was published by Hirsch et al. on behalf of ACC/AHA (American College of Cardiology/American Heart

Association) and collaborated by many other related organizations. This contains information on classification of levels of evidence and standards of their acceptance. The diseases included are lower extremity, renal, mesenteric and abdominal aortic aneurysms [37].

The American College of Cardiology Foundation (ACCF) and American Heart Association (AHA) jointly published a set of guidelines for diagnosis and management of patients with TA [38]. This contains the following:

1. Recommendations for imaging and detection/identification/evaluation of genetic syndromes, familial TA and dissections and bicuspid aortic valve and associated congenital variants in adults.

2. Estimation of pretest risk of thoracic aortic dissection.

3. Initial evaluation and management of acute thoracic aortic disease.

4. Surgical intervention for acute thoracic aortic dissection and intramural hematoma without intimal defect and history.

5. Physical examination of thoracic aortic disease.

6. Medical treatment of patients with thoracic aortic diseases, asymptomatic patients with ascending aortic aneurysm and symptomatic patients with TA.

7. Open surgery for ascending aortic aneurysm, aortic arch aneurysms, descending thoracic aorta and thoracicoabdominal aortic aneurysm.

8. Counselling and management of chronic aortic diseases in pregnancy, aortic arch and thoracic aortic atheroma and athero-embolic diseases.

9. Periprocedural and perioperative management.

10. Surveillance of thoracic aortic disease and previously repaired patients and employment and lifestyle in patients with thoracic aortic disease.

Several guidelines are being published by a variety of organizations within countries internationally. It is appropriate to evaluate these guidelines with respect to their usefulness in routine clinical practices. Ferket et al. in 2012 reviewed the guidelines published on screening for AAA during 2003–2010. Of 2415 titles, 7 were included in this study. These were USPSTF2005, ACC2005, NSC2007, CSVS2007, CCS2005, SVS1 of 2004, and SVS2 of 2009 [39]. Unfortunately, some of the more recent ones discussed above were not included. Some changes in the classification systems of ICD in different years could also affect evaluation.

There was consensus across the guidelines regarding one-time screening of elderly men to detect and treat aneurysms of larger than 5.5 cm in size. For smaller aneurysms and other target groups, prediction models and effectiveness analysis are needed.

The American Image Management (AIM) guidelines on diagnostic imaging, known as AIM, 2010, contain imaging protocols for various parts of the body using CT, MRI, PET, CTA, MRA and other imaging methods including proton beam treatment. These have also been published in parts as updated versions later in 2014 [40].

The American College of Radiology (ACR) has also published appropriateness criteria for AAA interventional planning and follow-up [43, 44]. It contains rating for appropriateness for planning pre-endovascular repair or open repair and for follow-up after these repairs with a note by experts. Best practice guidelines on clinical decision support systems have been published by the ACR and Radiology Business Management Association (RBMA) jointly. This contains evidence-based best practices related to all heath-care service components aimed at best patient outcomes. Other ACR guidelines are on the development of evidence tables for diagnostic studies, literature search process, non-traumatic aortic disease, procedure information like contrast used and PET and topic review process. All these appropriateness criteria (as they are called) follow a standard format containing explanatory notes by experts. Recently a study was conducted [41] in Sweden, to estimate the effect of AAA screening on disease-specific mortality, incidence and surgery. It was found that AAA mortality in Swedish men has decreased from 36 to 10 deaths per 100,000 men aged 65–74 years between the early 2000s and 2015. Mortality decreased at similar rates in all Swedish counties, irrespective of whether AAA screening was offered. It was mentioned that AAA screening in Sweden did not contribute substantially to the large observed reductions in AAA mortality and such reductions were mostly caused by other factors, probably reduced smoking.

The National Guideline Clearinghouse is a database for evidence-based clinical practice guidelines prepared by various organizations for comparison, synthesizes guidelines prepared by different agencies on the same topic for similarities and differences and serves as an electronic platform for exchanging information on such guidelines and is also a source of annotated bibliography database. Two of these deal with cardiovascular diseases [42].

2.3 Hospital compliance of ACR guideline on abdominal aortic aneurysm

Huber et al. collected NIS data for 1994–1996 [43]. Most patients were white males. Majority of repairs were done at large, urban and non-teaching hospitals. The hospital mortality rate was 4.2%. There was 32.4% incidence of complications. Home discharge rate was 91.2%. Bad outcome was experienced in 12.6%. Bad outcome was related to age, gender, complications and comorbidities (patient classifications) and hospital size and year of procedure. The authors concluded that outcome after open repair of intact AAA in US was good. However, only white males visiting the hospitals and procedures done only at large, urban non-teaching hospitals show skewed behaviour of AAA detection and treatment. There may be a certain degree of not falling in line with ACR guidelines in some respects. However, this is not clear from the results as only short-term data were selected and the methods used were unable to detect this.

The extent of compliance with long-term surveillance recommendations following EVAR and type B aortic dissection was found poor due to lack of coordinated approach. Cases of 204 patients (171 EVAR, 33 type B dissection) were evaluated. Of 171 EVAR, 100 were AAA, 45 TA, 12 TAA and 7 iliac artery and 7 proximal graft extensions. Medium follow-up period was 28 $\pm$ 10.5 months. Overall, 56% were lost to follow-up, and 11% never returned after initial hospitalization [44]. Lakhani et al. reported an increase in nonroutine radiological communications especially of critical finings in a tertiary hospital during 1997–2005 due to increasing compliance with ACR guidelines [45]. According to Benjamin et al. [46], compliance of the radiologist with hospital guidelines for nonroutine communication of diagnostic imaging results gave better outcomes in a general hospital. Such communications were required most for CT, followed by MRI and ultrasound.

Good correlation was found by Gilk et al., [47] between 2013 updated ACR guidelines on MR safe practices and the Joint Commission's Sentinel Event Alert No 39 on MR safety as the Environment of Care standards. About 90% of US academic emergency departments deviated from ACR guidelines on contrast practices for abdominal and pelvic CT imaging, as observed by [48]. According to Abramson et al., there are wide variations with respect to compliance on ACR guidelines by different hospitals [49]. Some reports on compliance of hospitals with ACR guidelines on fluoroscopy and CT were cited and discussed [50]. Quality assurance protocols, tracking exposure time and direct measurement of patient exposure time all based on ACR guidelines have improved compliance in reducing radiation exposure in some hospitals.

Besides these reports on some factors related to compliance of hospitals with ACR guidelines, many individual hospitals have reported receiving awards and certificates of ACR imaging compliance.

In general, there are no direct studies on the effect of extent of ACR compliance on aneurysm deaths. The findings discussed above only indicate the lack of compliance on certain aspects of ACR guidelines but nothing to connect them with aneurysm mortality. The importance of this study is evident from this research gap.

2.4 Frequencies of aneurysm diagnostic imaging by different modalities

Aneurysm is a chronic disease usually affecting people towards the end of their lives. This makes detection and intervention procedures highly risky. A majority of aneurysm patients do not report to the hospitals. Among those reported, repair procedure is not done on a good majority. It is notable that imaging helps proper diagnosis eventually leading to the reduction of mortality. Abdominal aortic aneurysm is most common with roughly 73% accounted, followed by thoracic aortic aneurysm. All others occur in very low frequencies compared to these. Although EVAR is promising, OAR is still the choice method, probably as the best method to deal with emergency and urgent admissions of ruptured aneurysms. In spite of other more promising methods becoming increasingly available, DSA is still the gold standard for diagnostic imaging. Such techniques like MRI and CT were used very rarely.

The data related to different types of aortic aneurysm admissions in US hospitals are given in **Figure 2**.

Out of a total number of 32,434 cases, elective admission dominated with 48.8% of valid data, followed by about 33.3% for emergency admissions. The latter is alarming as emergency admissions are usually associated with ruptured aneurysms

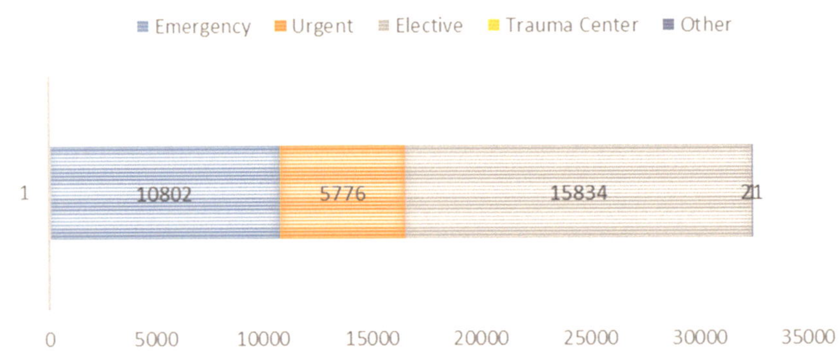

Figure 2.
Admission type of aortic aneurysm patients in US hospitals.

Hospital contexts		Medical imaging procedures				Total	P
		CT	MRI	US	DSA		
Admission type	Emergency	340	59	1084	9319	10,802	
	Urgent	53	10	469	5244	5776	
	Elective	73	20	2263	13,478	15,834	
	Trauma centre	0	0	2	19	21	
	Other	0	0	1	0	1	
Total		466	89	3819	28,060	32,434	<0.0001

Table 3.
Imaging frequencies using different methods of aortic aneurysm patients admitted in US hospitals.

and may lead to in-hospital mortality in spite of the best treatment given as it may be too late for any intervention to be successful. Urgent also is almost equally critical which accounted for about 17% of admissions. Emergency and urgent together constitute about 51% against 48.8% of elective admissions.

Different imaging methods may be used for different admission types. Thus more than 90% imaging was done with DSA in the case of emergency and urgent admissions compared to only about 79% for elective admissions (**Table 3**). Contrary to what was theorized, emergency plus urgent and elective admissions recorded almost equal 40–42% proportion of total patients for all imaging modalities. Overall, highest frequency (13,478) was observed for DSA in the case of elective admissions, and the lowest frequency of 10 was recorded by MRI for urgent admissions. On the other hand, US was highest in elective followed by emergency admissions. CT and MRI were highest in emergency followed by urgent admissions. Trauma centre and other admission types recorded very low frequencies to make any significant impact. Thus irrespective of admission type, DSA is the choice method followed by US.

This question is answered by reviewing research works in which two or more imaging methods are compared for their efficiency and effectiveness of aneurysm diagnosis, in which some specific aspect of the algorithms of one or more is enhanced. Several scientists have compared different imaging methods for diagnosis of aneurysms in which some algorithmic enhancements and support systems have been made for increasing their effectiveness and efficiencies of diagnosis. The parameters for efficiency are accuracy of diagnosis either by experimental comparisons of image readers or by relative quantitative or qualitative assessments. The measure of effectiveness is the relative merits of diagnosing some specific characteristics of the aneurysm under study like location, size, anatomy, etc.

This study utilized a series of processing methods on the NIS data, data mining techniques and statistical procedures to attain its goals. Data cleaning, recoding and extraction were used to arrange the raw data for the analysis. Statistical analyses such as frequencies, correlation, chi-square analysis, logistic regression and multinominal logistic test were applied. All of these different methodologies were used to analyse and process a big data set derived from multiple years from 2008 to 2012 and geographically collected from more than 4300 hospitals across the USA.

2.5 Objectives, variables and statistical analysis procedures

The NIS data set on different variables covering the period of 2008–2012 were used in this project. The variables required to fulfill different objectives are as given in **Table 4**.

No	Objective	Statistical tests applied
1	To study the relation between imaging modalities and in-hospital mortality among aortic aneurysm patients through US hospitals	Pearson chi-square test
		McNemar's test
		ANOVA test
		Logistic regression test
2	To compare in-hospital mortality of EVAR with OAR when different diagnostic imaging techniques are used in both cases	Pearson chi-square test
		McNemar's test
		ANOVA test
		Logistic regression test
3	To evaluate the effect of using ACR recommended imaging methods and extent of compliance on in-hospital mortality	Pearson chi-square test
		Gamma correlation test
		Logistic regression test
4	To determine among different patient characteristics and hospital context, those factors which can be used for prediction and thereby reduction of in-hospital mortality to desired levels	Logistic regression test
5	To determine among significant predictor factors, which type of diagnostic imaging performed is associated with in-hospital mortality	Multinominal logistic test

Table 4.
Relationship of objectives and statistical analysis procedures.

2.5.1 Data availability

Availability of the required data is a major factor in the ability to perform the above tests. In this project, all the required data are to be sourced from NIS data set. Hospitals may have not have given the cause of death properly. They may have automatically assumed that aneurysm patients died due to aneurysm only. Aneurysm as the specific cause of death may be absent. Even if it is possible to get data on a number of patients who underwent different repair procedures, records may not allow classification of repair procedures versus death data. A similar problem may arise with respect to imaging procedures also. Compliance percentage may not be indicative of a specific influence of ACR unless it is very high. At medium or low percentage values, the specific parameters on which there is compliance may also be important. Thus, the type of data available in NIS data set and its relationship with ACR guidelines is important. These are described below.

2.5.2 NIS dataset

There are two parts: the core file and the hospital file.

The core file has the data elements depicted in **Table 5**. The first core element of DXn and PRn deals with ICD-9 diagnostic and repair procedural codes, respectively. Other elements relate to mortality and patient classifications. The patient

Core file element	Variable in the study	Type	Description
DXn	Aortic aneurysm diagnosis	Nominal	ICD-9 diagnosis codes
DXCCSn	Comorbidities	Nominal	Clinical classification software
PRn	Interventional repair and imaging procedures	Nominal	ICD-9 procedure codes
DIED	In-hospital mortality	Ordinal	Died during hospitalization
AGE	Age group based on WHO standardization	Ordinal	Age in group at admission from 1 to 21 age groups
FEMALE	Gender	Nominal	The sex of the patient (male or female)
RACE	Race	Nominal	The race and ethnicity of patient
PAY1	Insurance type	Nominal	Indicates the expected primary payer
SOURCE	Admission type	Nominal	Source of admission to point of origin for admission or visit
LOS	Length of stay	Ratio	Length of stay from 0 day as same-day stays to greater than 365 days
YEAR	Year	Ratio	Calendar year (2008–2012)

Table 5.
The core file data element format.

classifications include age, gender, race, insurance type, admission type as source and the calendar year to which the data pertains.

In the hospital file in **Table 6**, information on location and type, bed size and geographical region are available. This is the core NIS file on hospital.

Results of a recent research by the authors are discussed here. ACR has nine rating scales of appropriateness criteria for different imaging methods and aneurysm types. For convenience of application for any imaging method and aneurysm type in our study, these were reduced to three appropriateness criteria by combining the same rating of different imaging methods and aneurysm types and making the ratings clearer. Hospital-wise data from NIS on mortality status (died/not died) to evaluate the effect of ACR compliance level on reducing mortality rate. The results showed that increasing levels of ACR compliance reduced mortality rates. More systematic research may be required for confirming the results. ACR appropriateness guidelines for diagnostic imaging have been developed by a large team of experts who examined available research works for the quality of evidence to prescribe these guidelines. The guidelines are reviewed and updated when new evidence becomes available. Hence, there is enough logic in contending that

Hospital file element	Variable in the study	Type	Description
H-LOCTCH	Hospital location	Nominal	Hospital's location and teaching status
H-BEDSZ	Hospital bed size	Ordinal	Hospital bed size
HOSP_REGION	Hospital region	Nominal	The hospital's census region was obtained from the AHA Annual Survey of Hospitals

Table 6.
Data elements in NIS hospital files.

compliance with ACR guidelines will improve the patient outcome especially on reducing mortality rate.

The details of the methodology and results are given and are discussed with the support of scientific evidence.

2.6 Effect of strictly and fully ACR compliant imaging procedures on in-hospital mortality rate

If compliance level is critical in determining mortality rate, the use of imaging methods in strict compliance with ACR should reduce mortality substantially. However, there can be variations among imaging methods to produce this effect. This aspect was studied, and the data are presented in **Table 7**.

CTA had a very few number of patients reported, and hence zero mortality obtained here is suspect. CT imaging of abdomen and pelvis as well as thoracic regions recorded similar mortality rate in the range of 10.5–12.0. The mortality rate was only 5.3% for US and was the lowest 2.6% for DSA. Based on length of stay, DSA was found undesirable in the earlier discussions. However, mortality rate itself is minimum for DSA, and this may be associated with a short period of hospital stay. All statistical tests were highly significant. Therefore, if ACR compliant procedures are used, DSA method is most effective followed by US in reducing mortality rate.

Earlier, in **Table 8**, mortality rate for different imaging methods (irrespective of ACR compliance) was presented. The mortality rates in both tables agree. Chi-square tests gave highly significant likelihood ratio and linear-by-linear values. Thus the model fitted better with predictors, and the relationship is strongly linear (**Table 8**).

Gamma test and other tests have relatively low negative value indicating a negative relationship between ACR compliance and mortality. Gamma = −0.328, which also indicates a strong degree of inverse correlation. Thus, the higher the compliance, the lower is the mortality rate (**Tables 2–12**).

ACR radiological procedures		**Died during hospitalization**		**Total**
		Did not die	**Died**	
CTA	Count	4	0	4
	%	100.0%	0.0%	100.0%
CT: abdomen and pelvis	Count	199	27	226
	%	88.1%	11.9%	100.0%
CT: thoracic	Count	224	26	250
	%	89.6%	10.4%	100.0%
US	Count	4619	259	4878
	%	94.7%	5.3%	100.0%
DSA	Count	31,881	865	32,746
	%	97.4%	2.6%	100.0%
Total	Count	36,927	1177	38,104
	% within ACR	96.9%	3.1%	100.0%

Table 7.
The effect of using strictly and fully ACR compliant radiological methods on frequencies of in-hospital mortality of aortic aneurysm patients in the USA.

Chi-square tests			
	Value	**df**	**Asymp. sig. (two-sided)**
Pearson chi-square	206.255[a]	4	0.000
Likelihood ratio	152.579	4	0.000
Linear-by-linear association	197.995	1	0.000
N of valid cases	38,104		

[a]Two cells (20.0%) have expected count less than 5. The minimum expected count is 0.12

Table 8.
Chi-square test results on effect of ACR compliant radiological procedures on frequency of in-hospital mortality among aortic aneurysm patients in the USA.

ACR compliance rating		Died during hospitalization		Total
		Did not die	**Died**	
Usually not appropriate	Count	4619	259	4878
	% within ACR compliance rating	94.7%	5.3%	100.0%
	% within died during hospitalization	12.5%	22.0%	12.8%
May be appropriate	Count	32,304	918	33,222
	% within ACR compliance rating	97.2%	2.8%	100.0%
	% within died during hospitalization	87.5%	78.0%	87.2%
Usually appropriate	Count	4	0	4
	% within ACR compliance rating	100.0%	0.0%	100.0%
	% within died during hospitalization	0.0%	0.0%	0.0%
Total	Count	36,927	1177	38,104
	% within ACR compliance rating	96.9%	3.1%	100.0%
	% within died during hospitalization	100.0%	100.0%	100.0%

Table 9.
Effect of ACR compliance levels of hospitals on frequencies of in-hospital mortality.

Compliance level	In-hospital mortality percentage
Usually not appropriate	5.3
May be appropriate	2.8
Usually appropriate	0

Table 10.
Mean effects of increasing compliance with ACR appropriateness criteria on in-hospital mortality rate of aortic aneurysm patients in the USA.

Accordingly, the odds relationship for ACR compliance with mortality rate is given by the following equation:

$$\text{Ln (Odds)} = -1.472 - 0.676 \times \text{ACR compliance rating}$$

As the equation will result in a negative estimate, odds for mortality decrease when ACR compliance of hospitals increase. Significant Wald test value indicates no interference of other predictors on the relationship (**Table 13**).

Chi-square tests			
	Value	**df**	**Asymp. sig. (two-sided)**
Pearson chi-square	92.255[a]	2	.000
Likelihood ratio	78.896	2	.000
Linear-by-linear association	92.252	1	.000
N of valid cases	38,104		

[a]Two cells (33.3%) have expected count less than 5. The minimum expected count is 0.12

Table 11.
Chi-square test results on effect of ACR compliance levels of hospitals on frequencies of in-hospital mortality of aneurysm patients in the USA.

Symmetric measures					
		Value	**Asymp. Std. Error[a]**	**Approx. T[b]**	**Approx. Sig.**
Ordinal by ordinal	Gamma	−.328	.032	−7.617	.000
N of valid cases		38,104			

[a]Not assuming the null hypothesis
[b]Using the asymptotic standard error assuming the null hypothesis

Table 12.
Gamma test results on frequencies of in-hospital mortality of aneurysm patients as affected by ACR compliance levels of hospitals in the USA.

Variables in the equation									
		B	**S.E.**	**Wald**	**df**	**Sig.**	**Exp(B)**	**95% C.I. for EXP(B)**	
								Lower	**Upper**
Step 1[a]	ACR compliance rating	−.676	0.215	9.909	1	0.002	0.508	0.334	0.775
	Constant	−1.472	0.417	12.472	1	0.000	0.229		

[a]Variable(s) entered on step 1: ACR compliance rating

Table 13.
ACR compliance rating and various constants values.

3. Discussion

The aim of this chapter is to describe whether the extent of compliance with ACR diagnostic and interventional imaging guidelines by US hospitals influences in-hospital mortality rates of patients diagnosed with different types of aneurysms. The findings were expected to provide predictors of mortality outcomes under a given set of patient factors and hospital contexts. The need for any change in the guidelines or practices to reduce aneurysm mortality rates could be identified and recommended. Preliminary results had confirmed that out of the six main aortic aneurysm types, abdominal aortic aneurysm (AAA) was the most widespread type. About 75% of all aortic aneurysms was either AAA or rAAA. Another 21% of aneurysms belonged to thoracic aneurysm (TA). Thus, AAA and TA are the two types of aneurysms of specific concern. Although rupturing almost ensures death, only 3.4% of patients reported with ruptured aneurysm of any type. If only these patients die, overall mortality rate should be around 3.4%. Now the question arises:

which imaging methods were more commonly used in the case of ruptured aneurysms? Based on the findings, no specific imaging method was chosen for ruptured aneurysms. However, it is not certain that most of the mortalities occurred in the case of ruptured aneurysms only. It is also not certain that any other imaging method would have reduced mortality of patients with ruptured or intact aneurysms. As is evident from the above results, imaging methods were related to mortality rates: DSA recorded the lowest rate. All other imaging methods recorded higher than 3.4%.

The objectives of the study were specifically verified using various tests appropriate to the specific objective. The objectives were to establish that imaging methods had distinct influence on mortality rates, to compare the two intervention procedures in interaction with the imaging methods, to evaluate the impact of compliance with ACR guidelines on mortality rates, to examine the scope of using any patient factor or hospital context as predictors of mortality rates and to assess which imaging method is associated with mortality rate as affected by any of the significant predictors. The study relied on diagnosis and procedure of only the ICD-9 coding registered in NIS data set. NIS data does not include all the sophisticated diagnostic imaging procedure codes. Differentiation of pre- and post-operative imaging is not available in ICD-9 codes and is not indicated in NIS data also. This study was limited to the study of most common aneurysms and not all.

Only 5 years' data were included in this study. A more detailed study may need to be done for firm conclusions. Compatibility between NIS data and ICD codes need to be tested by using ICD-10 instead of ICD-9 to verify whether compatibility improves by this. Although several works reported increasing use of CT and MRI, this was not reflected in a data set as recent as 2008–2012. Similarly, increasing use of EVAR compared to OAR was also not reflected. This needs further investigation. How far probabilistic estimates of mortality based on predictors will be closer to actual figures is not clear either from published works or from this study. This aspect needs further study by developing such equations and comparing actual with estimates.

There is enough evidence that hospitals are less than fully compliant with ACR appropriateness criteria. However, their number is not known. A survey of US hospitals to evaluate numbers of fully compliant, partially compliant and non-compliant hospitals needs to be done. The latter two need to be persuaded to fully comply with the ACR criteria.

4. Conclusions

Recognizing the high mortality rates in certain aneurysm conditions, factors related to this were examined. Imaging methods have an important role in diagnosis and treatment interventions. ACR has published appropriateness criteria for diagnostic imaging. It was contended that if hospitals followed ACR guidelines, it would improve diagnosis and in turn intervention procedure also. The research was aimed at this aspect to develop predictors for mortality due to imaging methods and intervention procedures. Patient characteristics like age, gender, race, comorbidities and insurance type for medical reimbursement and hospital contexts like size, location, geographical region, type and admission types were included as variables for the study. The basic variables were four imaging methods and their combinations with EVAR and OAR upon which the patient characteristics and hospital contexts were superimposed. NIS data for the period of 2008–2012 from more than 4300 US hospitals were used. After prescribed data cleaning procedures, net sample size of 38,263 patients was obtained for detailed study. Apart from descriptive statistics, ANOVA, chi-square, logistic multiple regression, McNemar's and gamma tests were used for dealing with different objectives of the study. AAA and TA were most frequent aneurysm types. DSA and US were the most frequent imaging methods. OAR was much more frequently used than EVAR. Age group, male, and comorbidities had distinct effects on aneurysm frequency. More patients went to urban teaching and urban non-teaching, large-volume hospitals for emergency and elective admissions and were supported by medical reimbursement schemes. However, none of these patient characteristics or hospital contexts had any effect on frequency-based ranking of imaging methods or intervention procedures.

Results supported the view that imaging methods have a distinct effect on mortality. DSA recorded lowest and CT recorded highest mortality. Out of the intervention procedures, EVAR had lower mortality than OAR. However, in combination, OAR with DSA as the imaging method recorded lowest mortality. There was a distinct effect of hospital stay on these mortalities due to imaging methods with longer than 10 days for any imaging method increasing mortality risk. Definite effect of ACR compliance was observed. With increasing compliance, mortality rate reduced and became zero with full compliance. Thus, improving ACR compliance and patients selecting only compliant hospitals will reduce aneurysm mortality significantly. Results of logistic multiple regression were used for the development of probability equations for mortality with imaging methods alone and in combination with intervention procedures. From a detailed analysis of patient characteristics and hospital contexts, age group and comorbidities emerged as the most important predictors of mortality probability. Other factors were less important as they provided inconsistent results.

Overall, imaging methods affect mortality, and increasing compliance with ACR appropriateness criteria reduces mortality considerably. Probability of in-hospital mortality can be predicted using models with imaging methods with or without intervention procedures and adding age and comorbidity as predictors.

Conflict of interest

None declare conflict of interest.

List of abbreviations

TA	thoracic aortic aneurysm
rTA	ruptured thoracic aortic aneurysm
TAA	thoracicoabdominal aortic aneurysm
rTAA	ruptured thoracicoabdominal aortic aneurysm
AAA	abdominal aortic aneurysm
rAAA	ruptured abdominal aortic aneurysm
EVAR	endovascular aortic repair
OAR	open aortic repair
CT	computed tomography imaging
CTA	computed tomography angiography
MRI	magnetic resonance imaging
MRA	magnetic resonance angiography
US	ultrasound imaging
DSA	digital subtraction angiography imaging

Author details

Abdullah Al Amoudi[1], Shankar Srinivasan[2] and Mohamed Yacin Sikkandar[1*]

1 College of Applied Medical Sciences, Majmaah University, Majmaah, Saudi Arabia

2 Biomedical Informatics Program in Rutgers-SHP's Health Informatics Department, NJ, USA

*Address all correspondence to: m.sikkandar@mu.edu.sa

References

[1] Aortic Aneurysm Fact Sheet. United States Centers for Disease Control and Prevention Web Site. 2014. Available from: http://www.cdc.gov/dhdsp/data_statistics/fact_sheets/fs_aortic_aneurysm.htm [Accessed: 25 March 2017]

[2] Nordqvist C. What is an Aneurysm? What Causes an Aneurysm? Medical News Today Web Site. 2014. Available from: http://www.medicalnewstoday.com/articles/156993.php [Accessed: 25 March 2017]

[3] Hsiang JN, Liang EY, Lam JM, Zhu X-L, Poon WS. The role of computed tomographic angiography in the diagnosis of intracranial aneurysms and emergent aneurysm clipping. Neurosurgery. 1996;**38**(3):481-487

[4] Six Dimensions of Quality. Alberta Bone & Joint Health Institute Web Site. 2012. Available from: http://albertaboneandjoint.com/services/measuring-for-success/ [Accessed: 25 March 2017]

[5] Prestigiacomo CJ, Sabit A, He W, Jethwa P, Gandhi C, Russin J. Three dimensional CT angiography versus digital subtraction angiography in the detection of intracranial aneurysms in subarachnoid hemorrhage. Journal of NeuroInterventional Surgery. 2010;**2**(4):385-389

[6] Villablanca JP, Jahan R, Hooshi P, et al. Detection and characterization of very small cerebral aneurysms by using 2D and 3D helical CT angiography. American Journal of Neuroradiology. 2002;**23**(7):1187-1198

[7] González-Darder J, Pesudo-Martı J, Feliu-Tatay R. Microsurgical management of cerebral aneurysms based in CT angiography with three-dimensional reconstruction (3D-CTA) and without preoperative cerebral angiography. Acta Neurochirurgica. 2001;**143**(7):673-679

[8] Forsting M. CTA of the ICA bifurcation and intracranial vessels. European Radiology Supplements. 2005;**15**(4):d25-d27

[9] Hoh BL, Cheung AC, Rabinov JD, Pryor JC, Carter BS, Ogilvy CS. Results of a prospective protocol of computed tomographic angiography in place of catheter angiography as the only diagnostic and pretreatment planning study for cerebral aneurysms by a combined neurovascular team. Neurosurgery. 2004;**54**(6):1329-1342

[10] Karamessini MT, Kagadis GC, Petsas T, et al. CT angiography with three-dimensional techniques for the early diagnosis of intracranial aneurysms. Comparison with intra-arterial DSA and the surgical findings. European Journal of Radiology. 2004;**49**(3):212-223

[11] Matsumoto M, Kasuya H, Sato T, et al. Can 3D-CT angiography (3D-CTA) replace conventional catheter angiography in ruptured aneurysm surgery? Our experience with 162 cases. Fukushima Journal of Medical Science. 2007;**53**(2):85-94

[12] Alamoudi AO, Haque S, Srinivasan S, Mital DP. Diagnostic efficacy value in terms of sensitivity and specificity of imaging modalities in detecting the abdominal aortic aneurysm: A systematic review. International Journal of Medical Engineering and Informatics. 2015;**7**(1):15-35

[13] Piotin M, Gailloud P, Bidaut L, et al. CT angiography, MR angiography and rotational digital subtraction angiography for volumetric assessment of intracranial aneurysms. An experimental study. Neuroradiology. 2003;**45**(6):404-409

[14] Biasi L, Ali T, Hinchliffe R, Morgan R, Loftus I, Thompson M.

Intraoperative DynaCT detection and immediate correction of a type 1a endoleak following endovascular repair of abdominal aortic aneurysm. Cardiovascular and Interventional Radiology. 2009;**32**(3):535-538

[15] Stavropoulos SW, Charagundla SR. Imaging techniques for detection and management of endoleaks after endovascular aortic aneurysm repair 1. Radiology. 2007;**243**(3):641-655

[16] Chung J, Kordzadeh A, Prionidis I, Panayiotopoulos Y, Browne T. Contrast-enhanced ultrasound (CEUS) versus computed tomography angiography (CTA) in detection of endoleaks in post-EVAR patients. Are delayed type II endoleaks being missed? A systematic review and meta-analysis. Journal of Ultrasound. 2015:**18**(2):91-99

[17] van Gelder JM. Computed tomographic angiography for detecting cerebral aneurysms: Implications of aneurysm size distribution for the sensitivity, specificity, and likelihood ratios. Neurosurgery. 2003;**53**(3): 597-606

[18] Sailer A, de Haan M, Peppelenbosch A, Jacobs M, Wildberger J, Schurink G. CTA with fluoroscopy image fusion guidance in endovascular complex aortic aneurysm repair. European Journal of Vascular and Endovascular Surgery. 2014;**47**(4):349-356

[19] Deák Z, Grimm JM, Mueck F, et al. Endoleak and in-stent thrombus detection with CT angiography in a thoracic aortic aneurysm phantom at different tube energies using filtered back projection and iterative algorithms. Radiology. 2014;**271**(2):574-584

[20] Wada K, Nawashiro H, Ohkawa H, Arimoto H, Takeuchi S, Mori K. Feasibility of the combination of 3D CTA and 2D CT imaging guidance for clipping microsurgery of anterior communicating artery aneurysm. British Journal of Neurosurgery. 2014; **29**(2):1-8

[21] Van der Vliet JA, Kool LJS, van Hoek F. Simplifying post-EVAR surveillance. European Journal of Vascular and Endovascular Surgery. 2011;**42**(2): 193-194

[22] Kamal DM. The Value of Duplex ultrasound versus contrast enhanced CT Scan in the follow-up of Endoluminally repaired Abdominal Aortic Aneurysm: A blinded study (Doctoral dissertation, McGill University). 2003

[23] O'Connell MK. Understanding abdominal aortic aneurysm progression through three-dimensional microstructure imaging. Vol. 682007

[24] Macedo TA, Stanson AW, Oderich GS, Johnson CM, Panneton JM, Tie ML. Infected aortic aneurysms: Imaging findings 1. Radiology. 2004;**231**(1): 250-257

[25] Thurnher SA, Dorffner R, Thurnher MM, et al. Evaluation of abdominal aortic aneurysm for stent-graft placement: Comparison of gadolinium-enhanced MR angiography versus helical CT angiography and digital subtraction angiography. Radiology. 1997;**205**(2):341-352

[26] Missler U, Hundt C, Wiesmann M, Mayer T, Brückmann H. Three-dimensional reconstructed rotational digital subtraction angiography in planning treatment of intracranial aneurysms. European Radiology. 2000; **10**(4):564-568

[27] Buhk J-H, Kallenberg K, Mohr A, Dechent P, Knauth M. Evaluation of angiographic computed tomography in the follow-up after endovascular treatment of cerebral aneurysms—A comparative study with DSA and TOF-MRA. European Radiology. 2009;**19**(2): 430-436

[28] van Rooij WJ, Sprengers M, de Gast AN, Peluso J, Sluzewski M. 3D rotational angiography: The new gold standard in the detection of additional intracranial aneurysms. American Journal of Neuroradiology. 2008;**29**(5):976-979

[29] Zhang L-J, Wu S-Y, Niu J-B, et al. Dual-energy CT angiography in the evaluation of intracranial aneurysms: Image quality, radiation dose, and comparison with 3D rotational digital subtraction angiography. American Journal of Roentgenology. 2010;**194**(1): 23-30

[30] Defillo A, Qureshi M, Nussbaum E. Indocyanine green videoangiography and intraoperative catheter digital subtraction angiography in the treatment of intracranial aneurysms: A consecutive series of 235 cases. Cureus. 2014;**6**(9)

[31] Pearl MS, Torok C, Wang J, Wyse E, Mahesh M, Gailloud P. Practical techniques for reducing radiation exposure during cerebral angiography procedures. Journal of NeuroInterventional Surgery. 2015;**7**(2): 141-145

[32] Sueyoshi E, Nagayama H, Sakamoto I, Uetani M. Carbon dioxide digital subtraction angiography as an option for detection of endoleaks in endovascular abdominal aortic aneurysm repair procedure. Journal of Vascular Surgery. 2015;**61**(2):298-303

[33] Wacker F, Valdeig S, Raatschen H, Meyer B. C-arm CT-an adjunct to DSA for endoleak classification in patients with endovascular repair of abdominal aortic aneurysms. RoFo: Fortschritte auf dem Gebiete der Rontgenstrahlen und der Nuklearmedizin. 2014;**186**(3): 247-252

[34] Mastracci TM, Cinà CS. Canadian Society for Vascular Surgery. Screening for abdominal aortic aneurysm in Canada: Review and position statement of the Canadian Society for Vascular Surgery. Journal of Vascular Surgery. 2007;**45**(6):1268-1276

[35] Walker TG, Kalva SP, Yeddula K, et al. Clinical practice guidelines for endovascular abdominal aortic aneurysm repair: Written by the standards of practice Committee for the Society of interventional radiology and endorsed by the cardiovascular and interventional radiological Society of Europe and the Canadian interventional radiology association. Journal of Vascular and Interventional Radiology. 2010;**21**(11):1632-1655

[36] Moll FL, Powell J, Fraedrich G, et al. Management of abdominal aortic aneurysms clinical practice guidelines of the European society for vascular surgery. European Journal of Vascular and Endovascular Surgery. 2011;**41**: S1-S58

[37] Smith ER. The Canadian heart health strategy and action plan. The Canadian Journal of Cardiology. 2009; **25**(8):451

[38] Hirsch AT, Haskal ZJ, Hertzer NR, et al. ACC/AHA 2005 practice guidelines for the management of patients with peripheral arterial disease (lower extremity, renal, mesenteric, and abdominal aortic): A collaborative report from the American Association for Vascular Surgery/Society for Vascular Surgery, Society for Cardiovascular Angiography and Interventions, Society for Vascular Medicine and Biology, Society of Interventional Radiology, and the ACC/AHA task force on practice guidelines (writing committee to develop guidelines for the management of patients with peripheral arterial disease): Endorsed by the American Association of Cardiovascular and Pulmonary Rehabilitation; National Heart, Lung, and Blood Institute; Society for Vascular Nursing; transatlantic inter-society consensus;

and vascular disease foundation. Circulation. 2006;**113**(11):e463-e654

[39] Taylor AJ, Cerqueira M, Hodgson JM, et al. ACCF/SCCT/ACR/AHA/ASE/ASNC/NASCI/SCAI/SCMR 2010 appropriate use criteria for cardiac computed tomography: A report of the American college of cardiology foundation appropriate use criteria task force, the society of cardiovascular computed tomography, the American college of radiology, the American heart association, the American society of echocardiography, the American society of nuclear cardiology, the north American society for cardiovascular imaging, the society for cardiovascular angiography and interventions, and the society for cardiovascular magnetic resonance. Journal of the American College of Cardiology. 2010;**56**(22):1864-1894

[40] Ferket BS, Grootenboer N, Colkesen EB, et al. Systematic review of guidelines on abdominal aortic aneurysm screening. Journal of Vascular Surgery. 2012;**55**(5):1296-1304

[41] Johansson M, Zahl PH, Siersma V, Jørgensen KJ, Marklund B, Brodersen J. Benefits and harms of screening men for abdominal aortic aneurysm in Sweden: A registry-based cohort study. Lancet. 2018;**391**(10138):2441-2447. DOI: 10.1016/S0140-6736(18)31031-6

[42] Diagnostic Imaging Utilization Management. American Imaging Management Web Site. 2010. Available from: http://www.aimspecialtyhealth.com/ [Accessed: 25 March 2014]

[43] American College of Radiology. Planning for Pre-Endovascular Repair (EVAR) or Open Repair of AAA. 2012. Available from: http://www.acr.org/Quality-Safety/Appropriateness-Criteria [Accessed: 11 May 2014]

[44] ACR Appropriateness Criteria® Abdominal Aortic Aneurysm: Interventional Planning and Follow-up. National Guideline Clearinghouse Web Site. 2010. Available from: http://www.guideline.gov/ [Accessed: 01 April 2014]

[45] Huber GS, Wang JG, Derrow AE, et al. Experience in the United States with intact abdominal aortic aneurysm repair. Journal of Vascular Surgery. 2001;**33**(2):304-311

[46] Kret MR, Azarbal AF, Mitchell EL, Liem TK, Landry GJ, Moneta GL. Compliance with long-term surveillance recommendations following endovascular aneurysm repair or type B aortic dissection. Journal of Vascular Surgery. 2013;**58**(1):25-32

[47] Lakhani P, Langlotz CP. Documentation of nonroutine communications of critical or significant radiology results: A multiyear experience at a tertiary hospital. Journal of the American College of Radiology. 2010;**7**(10):782-790

[48] Harvey HB, Alkasab TK, Pandharipande PV, Zhao J, Halpern EF, Salazar GM, et al. Radiologist compliance with institutional guidelines for use of nonroutine communication of diagnostic imaging results. Journal of the American College of Radiology. April 1, 2015;**12**(4):376-384

[49] Gilk T, Kanal E. Interrelating sentinel event alert #38 with the ACR guidance document on MR safe practices: 2013. An MRI accreditation safety review tool. Journal of Magnetic Resonance Imaging. 2013;**37**(3):531-543

[50] Broder JS, Hamedani AG, Liu SW, Emerman CL. Emergency department contrast practices for abdominal/pelvic computed tomography—A National Survey and comparison with the American College of Radiology Appropriateness Criteria. The Journal of Emergency Medicine. 2013;**44**(2):423-433

Chapter 3

Mycotic Aortic Aneurysms

Lucas Ribé Bernal, Lucía Requejo, Aida Ribes and Manuel Miralles

Abstract

Various studies have evaluated the possibilities of surgical repair of mycotic aortic aneurysms (MAAs). Open surgical repair has usually been accepted as the gold standard treatment of MAAs. The main concern is that it carries a significant mortality risk, varying from 20 to 40% in different studies, and a 5-year survival rate of 30–50%. The largest study of open surgical treatment of mycotic aortic aneurysms (MAA) was published in 2018, and consisted of 187 patients of whom open repairs were performed in 107 patients (57%). Most of the endovascular series conclude that endovascular treatment of MAA is feasible and an acceptable alternative treatment to open repair. Although endovascular repair might be a durable option for some patients, late infection-associated complications frequently occur and are often lethal. An overall analysis of this rare pathology, its different diagnostic modalities, treatment options, and prognosis are presented and discussed in this chapter.

Keywords: aneurysm, endovascular, aortic repair, infected

1. Introduction

Infected aortic aneurysms, also known as "mycotic aortic aneurysms" (or microbial arteritis with aneurysms) are most commonly caused by bacterial infections. Around 1% of arterial aneurysms may be associated with an arterial infection. Although the prevalence of mycotic aortic aneurysms (MAAs) is low, its clinical impact may be severe and represents one of the most difficult arterial diseases to treat successfully.

In the early nineteenth century, Jean Nicolas Corvisart coined the term "vegetation" as it resembled a cauliflower, describing organic lesions of the heart. In his monograph, presented in 1806, Corvisart wrote that he had observed six cases of valve disease with vegetations [1].

Some years later, in 1815, Joseph Hodgson performed some illustrations of ulcerating/perforating aortic valve endocarditis. He described the valve vegetations as "wart-like excrescences" using the term "fungus" in a patient who presented with an aortic root abscess. This report was probably the first to document peripheral embolization [2].

In 1852, a British physician, William Kirkes, described that fibrinous fragments of valve vegetations were found in the kidneys, cerebral artery, and spleen in patients presenting with fever, heart murmur, purple skin spots, and skin nodules (later called "Osler nodules" by Emanuel Libman). He described how these fragments could be detached from the heart valves, passed into the blood, and may be arrested in the aorta or its branches [3, 4].

The suggestion of an infection point of entry and transportation by blood flow was reinforced by a pioneering microbiologist, Edwin Klebs. In 1878, he suggested that cases of endocarditis were always due to an infectious organism [5].

The first complete description of an infected aneurysm was presented in 1885 by Osler. He presented the first broad report of this entity with a complete description of clinical and anatomical features of infective endocarditis as the cause of these arterial infections. The report included clinical features, anatomical location in the aorta, and cases of "ulcer formation and perforation of the aorta with production of multiple aneurysms" [6].

There were some other early reports that explained how infected aortitis was nearly always secondary to endocarditis [3, 5, 7, 8]. In another report published in 1923, a series of 217 patients with mycotic aneurysms was presented, showing that 86% of mycotic aneurysms were associated with infective endocarditis [9]. Although most infected aneurysms are due to bacterial infections, the term "mycotic," which is still misleading, is used to describe these aneurysms that arise after an inflammatory destruction of the arterial wall happens associated to arterial embolization. A wide variety of terminologies have been used to describe infected aortic aneurysms, although most of them have not received a great acceptance. Some of these include mycotic aortic aneurysms (MAAs), suppurative arteritis, septic aortic pseudoaneurysm (SAP), cryptogenic mycotic aneurysm, and microbial arteritis with aneurysms [10–13].

2. Etiology

Table 1 includes a previous classification of infected aneurysms (**Table 1**) [14]. The main etiology of MAAs is considered to be similar to that of arterial aneurysms and includes the following:

1. *Contiguous infection*: an infection localized in a determined area might extend and affect the arterial wall. This can happen after bone infections (osteomyelitis and vertebral infections), intraabdominal infections, abscesses, pancreatitis, and pancreatic pseudocysts. Arterial aneurysms have been described after surgical procedures such as a cholecystectomy, appendectomy, knee replacement surgery, or intestinal surgery [15, 16].

	Mycotic aneurysm	**Infected aneurysm**	**Microbial arteritis**	**Traumatic infected pseudoaneurysm**	**Contiguous septicemia**
Etiology	Endocarditis	Bacteremia	Bacteremia	Traumatic	Bacteremia
Location	Any vessel	Distal aorta	Aortoiliac	Femoral, carotid	Aortoiliac
Age	30–50	>50	>50	<30	>50
Sex	F > M	M	M	M/F	M/F
Incidence	Rare	Unusual	Common	Common	Unusual
Number	Multiple	Single	Single	Multiple	Multiple
Bacteriology	*Gram-positive cocci*	*Staphylococcus aureus, Escherichia coli*	*Salmonella*	*Polymicrobial*	

M: Male. F: Female.

Table 1.
Modified classification of infected aortic aneurysms according to Wilson et al. [14].

2. *Bacteremic seeding*: all arterial layers can be affected by bacteremic seeding, which may occur when there is a preexisting aneurysm, atherosclerotic plaque, or intimal injury. The intima is usually resistant to infection. Once it becomes diseased, bacteria may progress through it into other layers (media or adventitia). As the aorta is the most frequent site of atherosclerosis, it is also the most common location of primary arterial infection.

3. *Septic embolism*: embolization from heart chambers secondary to endocarditis (vegetations) can affect the intimal layer or vasa vasorum of vessels, leading to arterial wall infection and MAA formation. Embolization may occur in between 25 and 50% of patients with endocarditis, but only 1–5% develop symptomatic MAAs [17].

4. *Direct bacterial inoculation*: infected pseudoaneurysms after arterial injuries have become a common cause of mycotic aneurysms. The common femoral artery (CFA) is the most frequently affected vessel. Vascular trauma, gunshot or stab wounds to arteries, intra-arterial drug injection, and iatrogenic arterial injuries can produce a direct inoculation of bacteria into the vessel wall. Infected pseudoaneurysms resulting from drug injection using dirty needles may involve the CFA, external iliac, subclavian, and carotid arteries [18].

5. *Atherosclerosis*: MAAs may arise from preexisting aneurysms or atherosclerotic plaques.

3. Risk factors

Some important risk factors for development of MAAs include some of the following:

1. *Infection*: other sources of infection are the main cause of MAAs. Still today, the most common cause of MAAs is endocarditis, which explains more than 30% of cases [17]. The second most common infectious cause of MAAs is bacteraemia. Other infections have also been reported and associated to MAAs, including cholecystitis, pancreatitis, diverticulitis, urinary tract infections (UTI), soft tissue infections, and osteomyelitis.

2. *Arterial injuries*: previously described in etiology.

3. *Immunosuppression*: certain diseases and treatments may lead to impaired immunity states, including chronic corticoid use, alcohol abuse, diabetes mellitus, malignancy, chemotherapy, and severe neutropenia.

4. Epidemiology

Infected arterial aneurysms are relatively uncommon and can affect very different anatomical location and practically any artery. Depending on different studies presented in the literature, the most common sites for mycotic arterial aneurysms are the aorta and the intracranial cerebral arteries. Following Baddour publication in 2015, regarding an American Heart Association (AHA) statement report on infective endocarditis (IE) in adults, the most common site of mycotic aneurysms was the intracranial arteries, with an incidence of 1.5–5% of cases, and an overall mortality among those with IE of 60% [17]. Some other series have reported similar findings, with intracranial arteries being the most common site for mycotic aneurysms (especially the middle cerebral artery), with and incidence of symptomatic peripheral mycotic aneurysms of 1–5% [19].

Some other reports have published that the higher incidence sites of infected aneurysms are the abdominal aorta, followed by peripheral arteries (typically occurring at bifurcation sites), cerebral arteries, and visceral arteries, in descending order of frequency [20]. On the other hand, previous historical series have reported that the abdominal aorta was the second most common site of aneurysm infection, with the common femoral artery being the most common site [21].

Mycotic aneurysms of coronary arteries are rare, but have also been described. González et al. performed a review including 922 cases of definite infective endocarditis (IE), and reported a 2% rate of symptomatic peripheral mycotic aneurysms. In their review, 66% of mycotic aneurysms were intracranial (in the region of the middle cerebral artery) and 34% were extracranial [19].

With regard to infected aneurysms of the aorta, most reported series have less than 50 patients. Most series concur that the most common aortic location for infected aneurysms of the aorta is the infrarenal aorta, with a similar distribution of cases between the aortic arch and descending aorta.

One of the largest series involving MAAs presented 36 cases of aortic infection, with the following epidemiology data: infrarenal aortic aneurysm in 15 patients (42%), a suprarenal aneurysm in 3 (8%), a thoracic aneurysm in 5 (14%), and a thoracoabdominal (TAAA) in 13 (36%) [22].

A large multicenter European study was published in 2014, where data from 123 patients with 130 identified MAAs were analyzed. Similar epidemiologic findings were found, with infrarenal location being the most common (51%), followed by descending MAAs (28%), paravisceral (12%), multiple MAAs (6%), and arch MAAs (3%) [23].

Primary MAAs are a challenging and very complex vascular pathology. Although they represent a small proportion of patients within all aortic aneurysms, when left untreated, they almost always develop into rupture or lethal complications. Without treatment, there is a very high level of lethal complications, including aortic rupture, abscess formation, and sepsis [17].

5. Microbiology

With regard to bacteriological patterns in infected aortic aneurysms, there have been some changes in bacterial patterns depending on the published series decade. Some initial studies on aortic infection have presented their results confirming *Staphylococcus aureus* as the most common infectious cause, followed by *Salmonella* organisms [24]. A series of 17 patients with MAAs reviewed in 1998 presented *Staphylococcus aureus* as the most common responsible organism (29% of patients), followed by *Salmonella* organisms (24% of patients) [25].

This change in bacteriologic patterns was already observed in the early 1980s, when comparing those series from before 1965 and those from after 1965. Collected series from English language reported before 1984 (178 patients with 243 MAAs) showed that *S. aureus* was the most common organism (28% of cultures), followed by *Salmonella* (15% of aneurysms) and Streptococcus (10% of patients). This series reported how there was some alteration in the involved bacterial flora before and after 1965. A decrease in the incidence of *Salmonella* infections was seen after 1965 (10% compared with 38% prior to that date), as well as an increase in the incidence of *Staphylococcus aureus* (from 19 to 30%) [21].

Some current series have presented a much higher incidence of Gram-negative organisms compared with older series, with Gram-negative microorganisms seen in up to 35%

of cases. Different groups have described a higher incidence of aneurysm rupture and mortality in those patients with Gram-negative infections compared with Gram-positive organisms. Aortic aneurysms with *Salmonella*-related infections have been associated with a faster progression and higher risk of early rupture [23]. Recent series have published an increase in Gram-negative bacteria in MAAs, including *Salmonella*, *E. coli*, *Campylobacter*, *Enterobacter*, *Serratia*, and *Proteus* [23, 26]. Some of these series have reported even higher rates in Gram-negative bacteria (*Salmonella*) compared to Gram-positive [26–29].

Although bacteriologic patterns continue to evolve, *Staphylococcus aureus* remains the most common pathogen, reported in up to 28–71% of cases [21, 23]. Reports from North America and Europe have described Gram-positive Staphylococcus as the most prevalent bacterial responsible for MAAs. On the other hand, there are reported differences regarding infective organisms depending on the geographic area. Many reports from Asia have presented Gram-negative *Salmonella* species as the most prevalent infecting organism in MAAs [23, 27, 28, 30].

Depending on the different series, anatomical location, and geographic area, blood cultures have been found to be positive in 50–85% of patients, with organisms being able to be isolated from the aneurysmal tissue in 62–76% of patients [23–26].

Some reviews have related mortality with the type of microorganism involved in aortic infections. In a series of 22 patients who presented with aortic aneurysmal infection, mortality was 36% in those with *Salmonella*-infected aortas, and 82% in those patients with aortic infections due to other microorganisms. Some other series have reported similar findings in terms of lower mortality associated with *Salmonella*-aortic infections [23, 27–29].

6. Clinical presentation

Symptoms of mycotic aortic aneurysms are very commonly nonspecific in the initial development of the disease. Patients with MAAs often present with fever of unknown cause. Many series have reported fever as the most common presenting sign of MAAs. These patients with febrile illness frequently present with insidious onset, apathy, weight loss, and general malaise [24].

A high index of suspicion is of great importance in order to avoid delay in diagnosis, as the natural history of most of these untreated mycotic aortic aneurysms is fatality. The most common causes of death in these patients are lethal sepsis or massive hemorrhage due to rupture [24, 31].

A vast majority of patients are symptomatic at the time of diagnosis. Most groups have outlined rates of MAAs as symptomatic on diagnosis involving 93–100% of cases [28, 31]. One of the most common symptoms at the time of initial evaluation is localized pain. When present, pain is most commonly localized in the abdomen, chest, or back. Some groups have reported pain as the most common initial clinical symptom of MAAs, in up to 88% of patients [28, 32]. It has been previously reported that the classic triad of mycotic aortic aneurysms includes fever, pulsatile mass, and back pain. This triad has been described in around 40% of patients [31].

Other manifestations have been described associated to MAAs, including the following:

1. Rupture

Massive hemorrhage may be a sign of MAAs. Some reports have described aortic rupture in MAAs in 50–85% of patients [24, 28, 31].

2. Expanding hematoma

Intraabdominal retroperitoneal hematomas usually produce hypovolemic shock. In cases of infected aortoiliac or associated mycotic femoral aneurysms, superficial expanding hematomas might be seen.

3. Acute ischemia of the lower limbs

Embolization is a common clinical sign that increases limb loss and mortality rates.

4. Mesenteric ischemia

Infected pararenal of thoracoabdominal aortic aneurysms (TAAA) involving the superior mesenteric artery (SMA) may cause acute thrombosis of the SMA or embolization into the distal mesenteric branches, leading to intestinal ischemia.

5. Osteomyelitis

Infection of the aorta may produce contiguous infection of the lumbar or thoracic vertebra. Interchangeably, a bone infection affecting the vertebra may provoke an infection of an aortic aneurysm.

6. Gastrointestinal bleeding

Although rare, primary aorto-duodenal fistula may occur due to an infected aortic aneurysm, when erosion of the vessel affects the third portion of the duodenum. Erosion and rupture of a MAA into a gastrointestinal structure, such as the esophagus or appendix, have also been described.

7. Intraabdominal abscess

8. Hemoptysis, dysphagia, and hoarseness

Rupture of a mycotic thoracic aortic aneurysm or pseudoaneurysm, or aorto-bronchial fistula formation may lead to hemoptysis [33].

9. Heart failure

10. Compression

Constriction or displacement of nearby structures may be present due to MAAs.

7. Infected versus inflammatory AAA

Although inflammation is frequently associated with aortic aneurysms, the classical appearance of an AAA needs to be differentiated from aortic aneurysms that are infected. Also mycotic aneurysms need to be addressed and distinguished from a clinical entity known as "inflammatory aneurysms."

Approximately 3–10% of abdominal aortic aneurysms are characterized by increased inflammation surrounding the aneurysm. These inflammatory abdominal aortic aneurysms (IAAA) are typically differentiated from common AAAs by certain features. These include a classical description of periaortic inflammation as a white gleaming fibrotic surface with a thickened aneurysmal wall [34].

Other common features of IAAAs include major adhesions and fibrosis of close anatomical structures, such as the duodenum and ureters. This fibrosis commonly leads to indistinct retroperitoneal tissue planes on imaging studies.

The classic triad of IAAAs includes abdominal pain, weight loss, and elevation of inflammatory markers (CRP, ESR). Inflammatory aortic aneurysms are not associated with periaortic air or fluid and are not infected (tissue samples and blood cultures are negative).

8. Diagnosis

The diagnosis of mycotic aortic aneurysms might be very challenging. In the presence of fever, general malaise, and a pulsatile abdominal mass or aortic aneurysm in imaging testing, a MAA should be suspected and investigated. An early diagnosis of MAAs is essential as it is associated with a high rate of hemorrhage due to rupture and high rate of early sepsis and mortality. Once a MAA is suspected, the patient should be investigated with laboratory testing and imaging studies.

Various definitions have been proposed for the diagnosis of mycotic aneurysms, including clinical, laboratory and radiological features.

Most series agree that the definition of mycotic aortic aneurysm should include at least two of the following criteria:

- Fever, sepsis, or localized pain.
- Abnormal laboratory findings (elevated white cell count: WBC, C-reactive protein: CRP, or erythrocyte sedimentation rate: ESR).
- Positive blood or aortic tissue cultures.
- Specific radiologic findings, including: periaortic soft tissue air, fluid, or mass, saccular/multilobular aneurysm or pseudoaneurysm.

Some groups have used specific definitions to delineate mycotic aortic aneurysms, including all of the following: fever or sepsis, abnormal laboratory findings (elevated CRP or white cell count), positive blood cultures, and radiologic studies showing a false aneurysm (with or without stranding), periaortic fluid, or air around the aorta [35]. Common radiologic (CT and MRI) features of MAAs are an irregular aortic wall, a lobulated vascular periaortic mass, and peri-aneurysmal gas/soft-tissue mass/edema.

Although blood cultures may be negative in around 25–50% of patients, negative blood cultures alone are not enough to rule out infected aneurysms, and diagnostic testing should be completed.

Ultrasound scanning may be useful in diagnosing the presence of an aortic aneurysm, but it is not reliable for specific diagnosis of aortic infection. Digital subtraction angiography (DSA), besides being an invasive procedure, is not reliable for specific identification of features that suggest and diagnose an infected aneurysm.

Imaging studies for detection of MAAs include computed tomography scan (CT) and multislice CT angiography with 3D reconstruction, as well as magnetic resonance imaging (MRI). For many groups, MRI with gadolinium enhancement is becoming the noninvasive imaging modality of choice for the diagnosis of acute or chronic aortitis.

Nuclear medicine studies, including fluorodeoxyglucose-positron emission tomography (FDG-PET) and nuclear gallium scanning, are alternative modalities

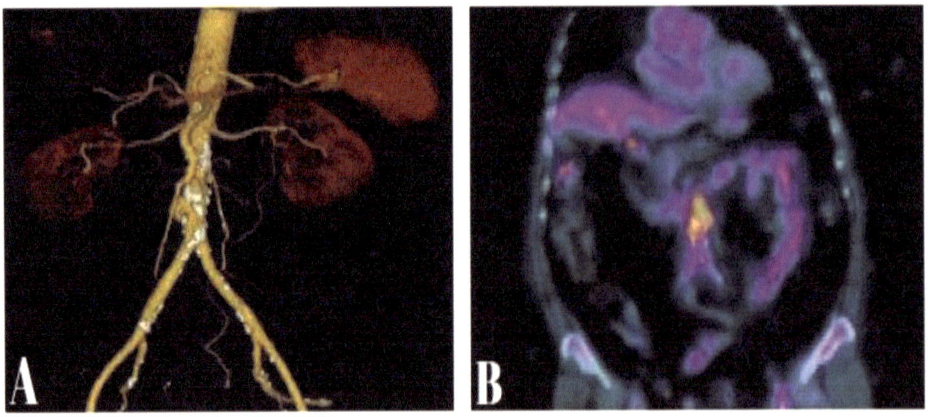

Figure 1.
CT scan showing a reconstruction of a distal infrarenal MAA (A). Fused frontal imaging of the contrast CT and FDG-PET scan showing highly elevated FDG uptake in the distal aorta (B).

	MAA grade I	MAA grade II	MAA grade III	MAA grade IV
Radiologic findings	1. A. ulcer or 2. A. mass or 3. A. pseudoaneurysm	Grade I and periaortic edema	Grade I and periaortic gas	Grade I and rupture (*)
Inflammatory markers (CRP and ESR)	+	+	+++	+++
Aortic tissue	—	+/−	+	+
Incidence	Rare	Very rare	Very rare	Very rare
Bacteriology	Absent	Present	Present	Present

MAA: mycotic aortic aneurysm; A.: aortic; CRP: C-reactive protein; ESR: elevated sedimentation rate; (*): contained or not; +: positive; +++: highly positive.

Table 2.
Ribé's proposal of new modified classification of MAAs.

for evaluating mycotic aortic aneurysms that are becoming increasingly useful. PET-CT testing has a very high sensitivity and both high positive and negative predictive values for aortic graft infection, and also provides important information in the diagnosis of mycotic aneurysms [35].

Current imaging studies have reported variable sensitivities regarding FDG-PET. Most series have published specificities of 88–100% for 18F-FDG PET and PET-CT for diagnosing active inflammation in arteritis (**Figure 1**) [35–37].

There are very few classifications regarding infected aortic aneurysms. The author would like to add a new modified classification of MAAs (**Table 2**).

9. Management of MAAs

9.1 Antibiotherapy

9.1.1 Recommendations

Various groups recommend vancomycin plus an anti-Gram-negative antibiotic (for coverage of *Salmonella* and Gram-negative microorganisms), including intravenous fluoroquinolone, ceftriaxone, and piperacillin-tazobactam. Results of blood cultures and tissue samples are monitored for hours or days, until a pathogen is correctly identified. Empirical antimicrobial therapy is maintained during this time, and reviewed once a pathogen is defined. Antibiotherapy should then be tailored to cultures and antimicrobial susceptibility [23, 24, 31].

In general, at least 6 weeks of intravenous plus oral antibiotics should be implemented. However, there are no data to support specific duration of antibiotic therapy. Several authors have advocated long-term oral antibiotics after hospital discharge for all patients undergoing intervention, especially those who underwent endovascular repair. If positive cultures are obtained from tissue samples, life-long antibiotic therapy should be considered [31, 32, 38, 39].

9.2 Surgery

9.2.1 Excision and ligation without arterial reconstruction

The aneurysm should be dissected back to normal aortic tissue. Once the aneurysm has been resected, the proximal aorta should be oversewn with a nonabsorbable suture, ligated 1–2 cm proximally, and possible omental coverage, to prevent blowout of the arterial stump.

9.2.2 Excision with immediate revascularization

In those cases where it is likely that the patient may develop acute ischemia after arterial ligation, immediate revascularization should be considered. Extra-anatomical bypass (axillobifemoral bypass graft) after aneurysm resection and stump closure has been traditionally used. Autogenous vein, antibiotic, and silver impregnated grafts are also used. Other reported options are femoral-popliteal deep veins, cryopreserved arterial allografts, and Dacron prosthetic grafts [39–41].

9.2.3 Excision with interval reconstruction

9.2.3.1 Hybrid repair

Some groups have described this technique of retrograde visceral revascularization (1, 2, 3, or 4 visceral vessels might be revascularized), followed by TEVAR/EVAR. The technique is performed through a midline laparotomy incision. When using the infrarenal aorta as the inflow vessel, a bifurcated 14 × 7 mm Dacron graft is prepared. Two side grafts (usually 6 mm Dacron grafts) are anastomosed to the lateral aspect of the bifurcated graft, to create the 4-graft retrograde bypass. Correct routing and fashioning of the grafts are crucial to avoid early graft thrombosis. The right branch (6–7 mm) is anastomosed to the right renal artery (RA). The right 7 mm graft would be anastomosed side-to-end to the coeliac axis (tunneled in a retropancreatic position). To avoid graft kinking, the left 7 mm graft is anastomosed in an end-to-side fashion to the SMA in a “lazy C” configuration [42].

9.3 Endovascular

Endovascular repair may be a suitable option for infected aortic aneurysms in high-risk patients, when open surgery mortality would be prohibitive. In cases of ruptured MAAs, endovascular repair may be an appropriate alternative, as a definitive treatment or until debridement and a final treatment may be performed. There is still ongoing controversy in the literature regarding the endovascular option as a main therapy or as an alternative [23, 30, 34, 39, 43].

Procedures are usually performed under epidural or general anesthesia, with open exposure of one or both common femoral arteries. In those undergoing TEVAR, cerebrospinal fluid (CSF) drainage should be considered in those patients with expected long thoracic segment coverage. Coverage of the left subclavian artery (LSA) is usually avoided unless completely necessary. Some authors have described aneurysm sac drainage after EVAR. The procedure is usually performed in a prone position. A 21-G needle is inserted into the aneurysm sac. Following dilation, a 14–16 Fr drainage catheter is used to aspirate and send the contents for microbiological analysis. Pryluck et al. consider that it might aid to decrease the infectious content of the aneurysm sac and effectively prevent late reinfection [44].

10. Prosthetic aortic infection

Although this chapter tries to focus on primary MAAs, infected aneurysms or pseudoaneurysms can also occur following prosthetic replacement of the aorta.

The incidence of prosthetic aortic graft infection has been described in 0.5–2% of cases, including both early and delayed-onset complications [45]. All these prosthetic graft infections are associated with high morbidity and mortality rates. As previously described in the chapter, different surgical techniques have been described for repair of infected MAAs and aortic graft infection. Removal of all infected tissue and infected grafts are essential for a successful result.

Plastic surgery-reassembling procedures have also been described for coverage of arterial tissue after reconstruction, especially after infections involving the ascending aorta, aortic arch, and descending thoracic aorta. These procedures involve musculocutaneous pedicled flaps using various different muscles (including rectus abdominis, pectoralis major, latissimus dorsi, and vastus lateralis muscles) [46]. The application of these vascularized muscle and omental flaps by plastic surgeons, in conjunction with cardiothoracic and vascular surgeons, might be an important alternative for an adequate management of these prosthetic aortic infections. Omental flaps have been previously described as the most common applied type of autologous flap for coverage of ascending aorta, aortic arch, and descending thoracic aortic graft infections. Other options for wound closure in cases of infected prosthetic aortic grafts with associated wound infection include different types of vacuum-assisted closure (VAC) devices [46].

11. Clinical cases

We present here a report of 3 cases of MAAs treated in our center, with a description of the procedural techniques and outcomes.

11.1 Clinical case description

The first patient (JGR) was a 72-year-old male with a medical background of smoking, who was evaluated for fever and general malaise. Physical examination revealed an expansive abdominal pulsatile mass, with pain on palpation. Laboratory testing showed elevation of elevated WBC ($22 \times 10^3/\mu L$), and inflammatory markers (CRP, ESR, and procalcitonin). CT angiogram revealed an infected infrarenal AAA, measuring 9.2 cm in diameter, with periaortic edema and gas (**Figure 2**). After cardiac, pulmonary, and renal evaluation, the patient was treated with an aorto-aortic silver-coated Dacron bypass graft. Blood cultures were positive for Staphylococcus aureus. After an uneventful recovery, he was discharged from hospital 10 days after surgery on long-term antibiotics.

The second patient (ABM) was a 66-year-old male with a medical history of chronic obstructive pulmonary disease (COPD), hypertension, and smoking. He was initially evaluated in the emergency department for hematochezia, fever, and abdominal pain. Physical examination showed a distended abdomen with an abdominal pulsatile mass. Laboratory testing showed markedly elevated inflammatory markers, including CRP and ESR. The patient presented sudden rectal bleeding and hypotension. Emergent CT angiography scan demonstrated a MAA at the level of the infrarenal aorta, with an associated primary aorto-enteric fistula (AEF) **Figure 3**.

He was taken to the operating room and had an urgent open aortic and small bowel repair. An aorto-aortic straight bypass graft, using a silver-coated-Dacron graft, was performed. Repair of the fistula into the jejunum was carried out with resection of the perforated bowel, and end-to-end anastomosis of a non-affected segment of jejunum. A Jackson-Pratt drain was left for 6 postoperative days. Blood cultures and aortic tissue sample were both positive for *Salmonella* sp. The patient was kept in the intensive care unit (ICU) for 5 days. After evaluation by the infectious disease team, he was discharged home on long-term antibiotics 16 days after the surgery.

He had a follow-up at 1, 6, and 12 months. His last CT scan showed no signs of aortic infection, without elevation of inflammatory markers on laboratory testing. His latest physical examination revealed no vascular abnormalities.

The third patient (RMS) was a 74-year-old male who was admitted with persistent back pain and fever. CT scan revealed a juxtarenal infected aortic aneurysm

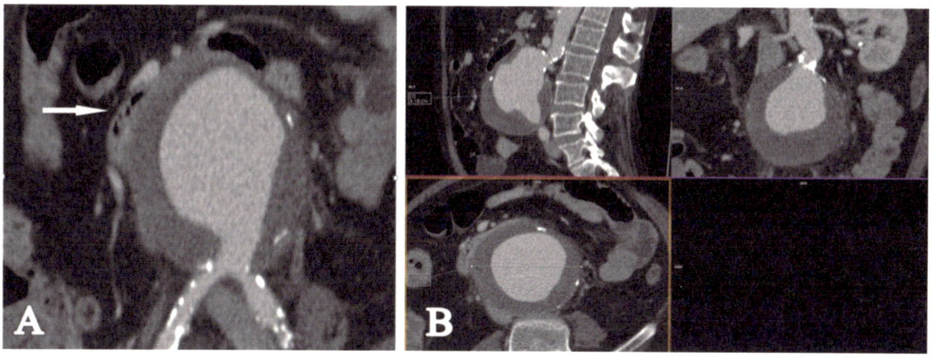

Figure 2.
Patient 1. Chest computed tomography (CT) scan presenting a 9-cm MAA in the infrarenal aorta. MAA compressing (white arrow) the duodenum (A). Sagittal, frontal, and sagittal planes (B). MAA: mycotic aortic aneurysm.

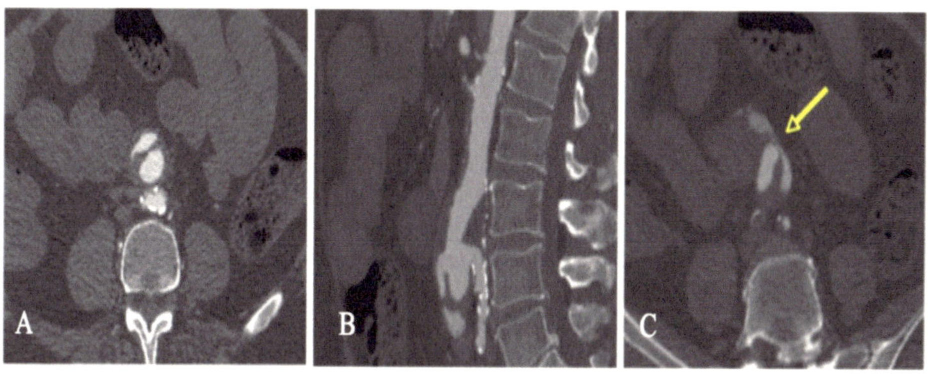

Figure 3.
Patient 2. Abdomen angiography CT scan showing an infrarenal MAA. Multilobular mass seen in axial (A) and sagittal (B) planes. Presence of an aortoenteric fistula (AEF) at the site (yellow arrow) of this MAA (C).

with gas within the aneurysmal sac, measuring 9 cm in diameter (**Figure 4**). Further preoperative MRI-imaging revealed spondylodiscitis at the level of the lumbar vertebra L3-L4 (**Figure 4**).

The patient was taken to the operating room and underwent an aorto-aortic straight rifampicin-bonded Dacron bypass-graft. Subsequent aortic wall tissue and blood cultures were found to be both positive for *Staphylococcus aureus*. Intravenous antibiotics were continued throughout the admission period and for 3 months after. After evaluation of the vertebral osteomyelitis by the orthopedic and microbiologist teams, he was discharged from the hospital 14 days after surgery on long-term intravenous (initially) and oral antibiotics.

Since 2011, we have performed in our center a novel hybrid repair in 2 cases of mycotic aortic aneurysms (MAAs), one of them a primary juxtarenal MAA, and the other one a suspected inflammatory infrarenal aortic aneurysm. This hybrid repair consisted in a two-stage procedure, performed within at least one-month difference, or once inflammatory markers and radiologic imaging studies had normalized.

The first stage of the procedure consisted in performing an open repair of the MAA, with interposition of a cryopreserved arterial allograft. This was done in 2 patients who presented with abdominal pain and a pulsatile mass on physical examination, with a CT angiogram that showed a contained ruptured aortic aneurysm in both cases. An aorto-aortic bypass graft using a cryopreserved arterial allograft was performed in both cases (**Figure 5**).

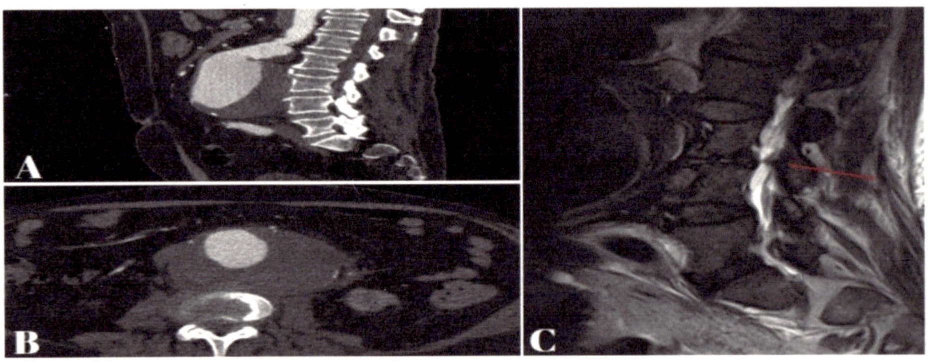

Figure 4.
Patient 3. CT scan revealing a juxtarenal MAA with gas within the aneurysmal sac (B), measuring 9 cm in diameter (A). Magnetic resonance imaging (MRI) showing vertebral osteomyelitis (spondylodiscitis) in a sagittal plane, with bone erosion (red arrow) at the level of vertebral bodies L3-L4 (C).

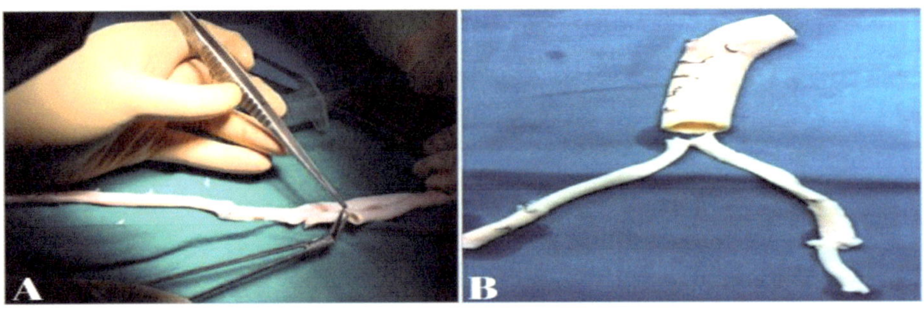

Figure 5.
Intraoperative images showing the surgical preparation of the arterial aortic cryopreserved allografts (A and B).

In the second stage, an endoprosthesis (Zenith® stent graft, Cook Medical Inc., Bloomington, Indiana, USA) was implanted just below the renal arteries, in the infrarenal aorta, 1 month after the procedure in the first patient. In the second case, an aortic endoprosthesis (Zenith Flex® stent graft, Cook Medical Inc., Bloomington, Indiana, USA) was deployed in the infrarenal aorta, sealing the inside of the cryopreserved allograft, 6 months after the initial procedure.

We believe that this alternative option might decrease the risk of rupture of the cryopreserved allograft anastomosis, which is a devastating complication of open repair of MAAs [23, 41].

12. Discussion

Treatment of aortic infection is still one of the most challenging situations for a vascular surgeon to confront.

Open extra-anatomic bypass revascularization combined with extensive debridement of all infected aortic and peri-aortic tissues, with excision of the infected aorta and oversewing of the non-infected aortic stump has been considered the standard treatment for aortic infection [22, 26, 31].

Open surgical options include the use of antibiotic-soaked Dacron grafts, cryopreserved aortic allografts, and biological bovine pericardial materials. The use of the superficial femoral vein (SFV)and femoral or popliteal vein segments have also been used as an alternative to in situ reconstructions in aortic infections [26, 32]. Revascularizations using vein grafts have the advantage of a potential lower risk of infection/reinfection. SFV as an autologous material has shown excellent performance in terms of long-term infectious complications. The main disadvantage is that vein harvesting is time-consuming. Another possible disadvantage of using the SFV is its diameter discrepancy with the aorta, and the possible limitation of vein length. These vein reconstructions are also functional and durable on follow-up over time [47–49].

Some groups have presented lower rates of recurrent infection and lower morbidity and mortality rates associated with rifampicin-soaked Dacron grafts compared to those with untreated grafts [35, 45].

Cryopreserved arterial allografts have the advantage of a higher resistance to infection, with low rates of reinfection. Techniques in cryopreservation have improved in the last decade, possibly contributing to better outcomes of revascularization using these allografts [35, 41, 50].

MAAs of the ascending aorta and aortic arch, without a past medical history of previous cardiac or cardiovascular surgery, are very rare. Macedo et al. reported an incidence of 2.6% of MAAs of the ascending aorta after a review of their more than 25-year experience with aortic mycotic aneurysms [51]. Descriptions of mycotic ascending aortic aneurysms or pseudoaneurysms in the literature are very scarce. MAAs of the thoracoabdominal aorta are also less common than those of the infrarenal aorta. Previous series have presented an incidence of primary infection of the thoracic and thoracoabdominal aorta affecting 0.7–4.5% of aortic aneurysms altogether [35]. Mycotic saccular, fusiform, and pseudoaneurysms of the ascending and descending thoracic aorta have been described in the literature. Repair of these aneurysms may be performed with different techniques, including cryopreserved arterial homografts, prosthetic antibiotic-soaked grafts, visceral debranching and endovascular stent-graft repairs, bovine pericardium patch grafts, and Dacron grafts with biological tissue coverage [35, 45, 52].

The largest series of mycotic aortic aneurysms was presented by Heinola et al. in 2018. This international multicenter study included 187 patients. In their series, 51 patients (27%) were treated with open prosthetic repair, 56 (30%) with a biological material, and 80 were treated with EVAR (43%). Overall, open repairs were performed in 107 patients (57%) in this group, making this the largest series up to date on open aortic repair of MAAs [32]. In their analysis, blood and/or tissue culture were positive in 43 (77%) cases, 33 (59%) were positive for non-*Salmonella* infection, and 10 (18%) were positive for *Salmonella* species. The most common registered bacterium on cultures was *Staphylococcus aureus* (27%). It presented a thirty-day survival of 95% (n = 53) and 90-day survival of 91% (n = 51). The overall treatment-related mortality was 9% (n = 5) [32].

The second largest study to date of open surgical treatment of mycotic aortic aneurysms (MAAs) was published in 2014 by Lin et al., including a group of 77 patients. In this study group, the in-hospital mortality rate was 10% (8/77) for patients who underwent open repair and 25% (2/8) for patients who underwent EVAR [27].

The first report of endovascular aneurysm repair of a MAA was reported in 1998 by Semba et al. They reported no postoperative complications from persistent bacteraemia after a 24-month follow up, without postoperative mortality [53]. Since then, there have been various case reports and series of cases describing EVAR and TEVAR for the treatment of ruptured aortic aneurysms and MAAs and their outcomes [23, 30, 34, 38, 39, 53]. These series report favorable results for EVAR/TEVAR for MAAs, providing a less invasive procedure with low early mortality rates [23, 30, 33, 34, 39, 53].

Kan et al. performed a systematic review of outcome after EVAR for the treatment of mycotic aortic aneurysms in 2007. They presented a life-time analysis, which reported a 30-day survival rate of 89% +/− 4% and a 2-year survival rate of 82% +/−5.8%. They performed a multivariate logistic regression analysis, which showed that only ruptured aneurysms and fever were significant predictors of persistent infection in EVAR after MAAs [38].

The largest series to date on endovascular treatment of MAAs was reported in 2018 by Heinola et al. This multicenter-group reported 187 MAAs treated in 6 different European countries between 2006 and 2016 [32]. Another previous large series on endovascular treatment of MAAs was reported in 2012 by Sedivy et al. This series included 32 patients, treated during a 15-year period. In this series, 81% of patients survived the 30-day postoperative period. A total of 50% survived after 1-year follow-up and 40% survived after a 3-year follow-up [50]. **Table 3** includes the most important series regarding MAAs (**Table 3**) [22–32, 35, 38–41, 54].

Although some of these modern series present promising results, with lower 30-day mortality for endovascular treatments compared to open surgery, the risk of persistent infection and late complications might be higher. Some concerns are present in modern literature regarding endovascular repair, as there are still no long-term follow-up of these series and there is still an ongoing controversy and debate regarding placing a stent-graft in a tissue (aorta) that is still infected.

For some complex thoracoabdominal aortic aneurysms (TAAAs), therapeutic options may be scarce. In those cases of symptomatic mycotic TAAAs, there may not be enough time to create fenestrated/branched custom-made endovascular stent-grafts. In order to avoid the high morbidity and mortality rates associated with total open surgical repair of these mycotic TAAAs, some groups have advocated for the performance of a hybrid aortic repair.

This hybrid repair of type I, II, and III TAAAs consists in performing a visceral artery debranching with retrograde revascularization, followed by the implantations of a thoracoabdominal endovascular stent-graft [42, 55, 56].

Contrary to what happens in the infrarenal abdominal aorta, extra-anatomic bypasses are very exceptionally used to repair primary MAAs of the thoracic and

Series	Year	Number patients	Technique	Mortality (30-day)
Moneta	1998	17	Open	23%
Soravia-Dunand	1999	10	Open	57%
Oderich	2001	43	Open	21%
Müller	2001	33	Open	36%
Fillmore	2003	10	Open	40%
Kyriakides	2004	15	Open	26%
Dubois	2010	44	Open	18.2%
Kan	2010	41	Open (n = 21)	4.8%
			EVAR (n = 20)	5%
Yu	2011	53	Open	23%
Weis-Müller	2011	36	Open	33%
Uchida	2012	23	Open	5%
Sedivy	2012	32	EVAR-TEVAR	18.8%
Huang	2014	43	Open (n = 29)	20%
			EVAR (n = 11)	9%
Lin	2014	109	Open (n = 77)	10%
			EVAR (n = 8)	25%
Sörelius	2014	123	EVAR-TEVAR	9%
Touma	2014	16	Open-Allograft	28%
Sörelius	2016	132	Open (n = 62)	26%
			EVAR (n = 70)	14%
Luo	2017	40	EVAR-TEVAR	10%
Corvera	2018	17	Open-Allograft	6%
Heinola	2018	187	Open (n = 51) EVAR (n = 80) Allograft (n = 56)	5%

Open, open surgical repair; EVAR, endovascular aneurysm repair; TEVAR, thoracic endovascular aneurysm repair.

Table 3.
Largest modern series of mycotic aortic aneurysms (MAAs).

thoracoabdominal aorta, or graft infections on those sites. Patients with mycotic aneurysms of the ascending aorta or arch may present with different signs and symptoms, including persistent fever, fatigue, chest or back pain, dyspnea, pleural effusion, and hypovolemic shock in cases of mycotic aortic rupture [57].

MAAs have also reported following heart transplantation and different cardiac surgical procedures. Bacterial, viral, fungal, and protozoal infections have been described after cardiac transplantation, understanding that these patients under immunosuppressive medication are at risk of mycotic aneurysm formation [58]. In cases of ascending, arch, or descending thoracic mycotic aneurysms associated with severe mediastinitis, surgical techniques for aortic repair include cryopreserved arterial homografts, repair with deep or superficial femoral veins, coverage with the use of the greater omentum, creation of pedicled muscular flaps for arterial coverage, tissue debridement, and sternal re-closure [45, 57, 58].

We described in this chapter 2 cases of a novel hybrid repair of MAAs, including a staged hybrid procedure, with a first stage including resection of the infected aneurysm and repair with an aortic cryopreserved arterial allograft, followed by a second procedure (once inflammatory markers have decreased and radiologic features have normalized) consisting of an aortic stent-graft. We believe that this option might minimize the risk of cryopreserved allograft rupture that has been previously described in the literature in cases of MAAs. Although there are no reports describing this technique, we consider that this might be a feasible alternative to prevent the risk of aortic rupture.

Long-term surveillance, including physical examination, laboratory assessment of inflammatory markers, and imaging studies (incorporating CT angiogram and FDG-PET or PET-CT) are critical for evaluation of possible complications and prompt decision in case of reinfections.

13. Conclusions

Treatment of mycotic aortic aneurysms (MAAs) remains a real challenge in modern vascular surgery. There are currently different treatment options, with an immense improvement in endovascular techniques and devices. Despite the fact of technological and endovascular improvements, this complex pathology is still associated with high morbidity and mortality rates. An early diagnosis and interventional procedure (open, hybrid, or endovascular repair) and aggressive antibiotic therapy are essential to improve outcomes.

Author details

Lucas Ribé Bernal*, Lucía Requejo, Aida Ribes and Manuel Miralles
University Hospital Le Fe, Valencia, Spain

*Address all correspondence to: lucasribemd@gmail.com

References

[1] Corvisart JN. Essai sur les Maladies et les Lesions Organique du Coeur et des Gros Vaisseaux (An Essay on the Organic Diseases and Lesions of the Heart and Great Vessels. Translated by J. Gates. Boston: Bradford and the Read; 1812). Paris: Mequigon-Marvis; 1806

[2] Hodgson J. A Treatise on the Diseases or Arteries and Veins. London: T. Underwood; 1815

[3] Kirkes WS. On some of the principal effects resulting from the detachment of fibrinous deposits from the interior the heart, and their mixture with the circulating blood. Medico-Chirurgical Transactions. 1852;**35**:281-324

[4] Libman E. A study of the endocardial lesions of subacute bacterial endocarditis. The American Journal of the Medical Sciences. 1912;**144**:313-327

[5] Ellis H. Edwin Klebs: Discoverer of the bacillus of diphtheria. British Journal of Hospital Medicine. 2013;**74**(11):641

[6] Osler W. The Gulstonian lectures on malignant endocarditis. British Medical Journal. 1885;**1**:467-470

[7] Rodis E, Yakirevich V, Almog C, Michaeli D, Vidne BA. Complicated infective endocarditis: Surgical treatment. The Journal of Cardio-vascular Surgery. 1985;**26**(1):64-66

[8] Osler W. On Some Points in the Etiology and Pathology of Ulcerative Endocarditis. Vol. 1. J.W. Kolckmann; 1881. pp. 341-346

[9] Stengel A, Wolferth CC. Mycotic (bacterial) aneurysms of intravascular origin. Archives of Internal Medicine. 1923;**31**:537-554

[10] Jarrett F, Darling RC, Mundth ED, Austen WG. Experience with infected aneurysms of the abdominal aorta. Archives of Surgery. 1975;**110**(11):1281-1286

[11] Blum L, Keefer EB. Cryptogenic mycotic aneurysm. Annals of Surgery. 1962;**155**:398-405

[12] Crane A. Primary multilocular mycotic aneurysm of the aorta. Archives of Pathology. 1937;**24**:634-641

[13] Benett DE. Primary mycotic aneurysms of the aorta. Report of case and review of the literature. Archives of Surgery. 1967;**94**(6):758-765

[14] Wilson SE, Van Wagenen P, Passaro E. Arterial infection. Current Problems in Surgery. 1978;**15**(9):1-89

[15] Mazzalai F, Ragazzi R, Iurilli V, Toniato A, Da Giau G, Ballotta E. Pseudomonas aeruginosa-infected infrarenal abdominal aorta pseudoaneurysm secondary to laparoscopic colorectal surgery: Failure of endovascular stent graft treatment after primary open repair failed. Canadian Journal of Surgery. 2009;**52**(5):E193-E194

[16] Woo SB, Cheng LC, Wong WC. Mycotic aortic aneurysm following treatment of pyogenic vertebral osteomyelitis. Asian Cardiovascular & Thoracic Annals. 2006;**14**(5):e102-e105

[17] Baddour LM, Wilson W, Bayer A, Fowler V, Tleyjeh I, Rybak MJ, et al. Infective endocarditis in adults: Diagnosis, antimicrobial therapy, and management of complications: A scientific statement for healthcare professionals from the American Heart Association. Circulation. 2015;**132**(15):1435-1486

[18] Stevenson RP, Semple C, Hussey K, McGovern J, Stuart WP, Kingsmore DB. Changes in the demographics of intravenous drug users with

mycotic common femoral artery pseudoaneurysm as a consequence of self-injection does not influence outcome following emergency ligation. Vascular. 2017;**25**(5):520-524

[19] González I, Sarriá C, López J, Vilacosta I, San Román A, Olmos C, et al. Symptomatic peripheral mycotic aneurysms due to infective endocarditis: A contemporary profile. Medicine. 2014;**93**(1):42-52

[20] Lee WK, Mossop PJ, Little AF, Fitt GJ, Vrazas JI, Hoang JK, et al. Infected (mycotic) aneurysms: Spectrum of imaging appearances and management. Radiographics. 2008;**28**(7):1853-1868

[21] Brown SL, Busuttil RW, Baker JD, Machleder HI, Moore WS, Barker WF. Bacteriologic and surgical determinants of survival in patients with mycotic aneurysms. Journal of Vascular Surgery. 1984;**1**(4):541-547

[22] Weis-Müller BT, Rascanu C, Sagban A, Grabitz K, Godehardt E, Sandmann W. Single-center experience with open surgical treatment of 36 infected aneurysms of the thoracic, thoracoabdominal, and abdominal aorta. Annals of Vascular Surgery. 2011;**25**(8):1020-1025

[23] Sörelius K, Mani K, Björck M, Sedivy P, Wahlgren CM, Taylor P, et al. Endovascular treatment of mycotic aortic aneurysms: A European multicenter study. Circulation. 2014;**130**(24):2136-2142

[24] Müller BT, Wegener O, Grabitz K, Pillny M, Thomas L, Sandmann W. Mycotic aneurysms of the thoracic and abdominal aorta and iliac arteries: Experience with anatomic and extra-anatomic repair in 33 cases. Journal of Vascular Surgery. 2001;**33**:106-113

[25] Moneta GL, Taylor LM Jr, Yeager RA, Edwards JM, Nicoloff AD, McConnell DB, et al. Surgical treatment of infected aortic aneurysm. American Journal of Surgery. 1998;**175**(5):396-399

[26] Dubois M, Daenens K, Houthoofd S, Peetermans WE, Fourneau I. Treatment of mycotic aneurysms with involvement of the abdominal aorta: Single-centre experience in 44 consecutive cases. European Journal of Vascular and Endovascular Surgery. 2010;**40**(4):450-456

[27] Lin CH, Hsu RB. Primary infected aortic aneurysm: Clinical presentation, pathogen, and outcome. Acta Cardiologica Sinica. 2014;**30**(6):514-521

[28] Yu SY, Hsieh HC, Ko PJ, Huang YK, Chu JJ, Lee CH. Surgical outcome for mycotic aortic and iliac aneurysm. World Journal of Surgery. 2011;**35**(7):1671-1678

[29] Hsu RB, Chang CI, Wu IH, Lin FY. Selective medical treatment of infected aneurysms of the aorta in high risk patients. Journal of Vascular Surgery. 2009;**49**(1):66-70

[30] Huang YK, Chen CL, Lu MS, Tsai FC, Lin PL, Wu CH, et al. Clinical, microbiologic, and outcome analysis of mycotic aortic aneurysm: The role of endovascular repair. Surgical Infections. 2014;**15**(3):290-298

[31] Oderich GS, Panneton JM, Bower TC, Cherry KJ Jr, Rowland CM, Noel AA, et al. Infected aortic aneurysms: Aggressive presentation, complicated early outcome, but durable results. Journal of Vascular Surgery. 2001;**34**(5):900-908

[32] Heinola I, Sörelius K, Wyss TR, Eldrup N, Settembre N, Setacci C, et al. Open repair of mycotic abdominal aortic aneurysms with biological grafts: An international Multicenter study. Journal of the American Heart Association. 2018;7(12):1-9

[33] Ribé L, Río J, Portero JL, Reparaz L. Late survival after endovascular repair of an *Aortobronchial fistula*. EJVES Extra. 2010;**19**(2):e22-e24

[34] Stone WM, Fankhauser GT, Bower TC, Oderich GS, Oldenburg WA, Kalra M, et al. Comparison of open and endovascular repair of inflammatory aortic aneurysms. Journal of Vascular Surgery. 2012;**56**(4):951-955

[35] Corvera JS, Blitzer D, Copeland H, Murphy D, Hess PJ Jr, Pillai ST, et al. Repair of thoracic and thoracoabdominal mycotic aneurysms and infected aortic grafts using allograft. The Annals of Thoracic Surgery. 2018;**106**(4):1129-1135

[36] Soussan M, Nicolas P, Schramm C, Katsahian S, Pop G, Fain O, et al. Management of large-vessel vasculitis with FDG-PET: A systematic literature review and meta-analysis. Medicine. 2015;**94**(14):e622

[37] Murakami M, Morikage N, Samura M, Yamashita O, Suehiro K, Hamano K. Fluorine-18-fluorodeoxyglucose positron emission tomography-computed tomography for diagnosis of infected aortic aneurysms. Annals of Vascular Surgery. 2014;**28**(3):575-578

[38] Kan CD, Lee HL, Luo CY, Yang YJ. The efficacy of aortic stent grafts in the management of mycotic abdominal aortic aneurysm-institute case management with systemic literature comparison. Annals of Vascular Surgery. 2010;**24**(4):433-440

[39] Sörelius K, Wanhainen A, Furebring M, Björck M, Gillgren P, Mani K. Nationwide study of the treatment of mycotic abdominal aortic aneurysms comparing open and endovascular repair. Circulation. 2016;**134**(23):1822-1832

[40] Kyriakides C, Kan Y, Kerle M, Cheshire NJ, Mansfield AO, Wolfe JH. 11-year experience with anatomical and extra-anatomical repair of mycotic aortic aneurysms. European Journal of Vascular and Endovascular Surgery. 2004;**27**(6):585-589

[41] Touma J, Cochennec F, Parisot J, Fialaire Legendre A, Becquemin JP, Desgranges P. In situ reconstruction in native and prosthetic aortic infections using cryopreserved arterial allografts. European Journal of Vascular and Endovascular Surgery. 2014;**48**(3):292-299

[42] Ribé L, Gibbs RG, Jenkins M, Wolfe JHN. Visceral and arch hybrid aortic repair for thoracoabdominal aneurysms. In: Greenhalgh RM, editor. Vascular and Endovascular Challenges Update. London, UK: Biba Medical; 2013. pp. 127-136. ISBN: 978-0-9570419-1-2

[43] Bernal LR, Portero JL, Vila M, Ruiz DF, Reparaz LM. Hemoptysis caused by a left subclavian pseudoaneurysm: Endovascular solution for a challenging case. Vascular. 2013;**21**(3):159-162

[44] Pryluck DS, Kovacs S, Maldonado TS, Jacobowitz GR, Adelman MA, Charles HC, et al. Percutaneous drainage of aortic aneurysm sac abscesses following endovascular aneurysm repair. Vascular and Endovascular Surgery. 2010;**44**(8):701-707

[45] Gebhard C, Biaggi P, Sthli BE, Schwarz U, Felix C, Falk V. Complete graft dehiscence 8 months after repair of acute type A aortic dissection. European Heart Journal Acute Cardiovascular Care. 2013;**2**(1):72-76

[46] Frautschi RS, Bassiri Gharb B, Duong MM, Gurunluoglu R, Papay F, Zins JE, et al. The cardioplastic approach to the treatment of infected aortic grafts. Annals of Plastic Surgery. 2017;**79**(2):221-225

[47] Chervu A, Moore WS, Gelabert HA, Colburn MD, Chvapil M. Prevention of graft infection by use of prosthesis bonded with rifampin/collagen release system. Journal of Vascular Surgery. 1991;**14**:521-525

[48] Daenens K, Fourneau I, Nevelsteen A. Ten-year experience in autogenous reconstruction with the femoral vein in the treatment of aortofemoral prosthetic infection. European Journal of Vascular and Endovascular Surgery. 2003;**25**:240-245

[49] Czerny M, von Allmen R, Opfermann P, et al. Seft-made pericardial tube graft; a new surgical concept for treatment of graft infections after thoracic and abdominal aortic procedures. The Annals of Thoracic Surgery. 2011;**92**:1657-1662

[50] Ben Ahmed S, Louvancourt A, Daniel G, Combe P, Duprey A, Albertini JN, et al. Cryopreserved arterial allografts for in situ reconstruction of abdominal aortic native or secondary graft infection. Journal of Vascular Surgery. 2018;**67**(2):468-477

[51] Macedo TA, Stanson AW, Oderich GS, Johnson CM, Panneton JM, Tie ML. Infected aortic aneurysms: Imaging findings. Radiology. 2004;**231**:250-257

[52] Mukherjee JT, Nautiyal A, Labib SB. Mycotic aneurysms of the ascending aorta in the absence of endocarditis. Texas Heart Institute Journal. 2012;**39**(5):692-695

[53] Semba CP, Sakai T, Slonim SM, Razavi MK, Kee ST, Jorgensen MJ, et al. Mycotic aneurysms of the thoracic aorta: Repair with use of endovascular stent-grafts. Journal of Vascular and Interventional Radiology. 1998;**9** (1 Pt 1):33-40

[54] Sedivy P, Spacek M, El Samman K, Belohlavek O, Mach T, Jindrak V, et al. Endovascular treatment of infected aortic aneurysms. European Journal of Vascular and Endovascular Surgery. 2012;**44**(4):385-394

[55] Antoniou GA, El Sakka K, Hamady M, Wolfe JH. Hybrid treatment of complex aortic arch disease with supra-aortic debranching and endovascular stent graft repair. European Journal of Vascular and Endovascular Surgery. 2010;**39**(6):683-690

[56] Jaffer U, Gibbs R. Mycotic thoracoabdominal aneurysms. Annals of Cardiothoracic Surgery. 2012;**1**(3):417-425

[57] Masuda S, Takeuchi N, Takada M, Fujita K, Nishibori Y, Maruyama T. Ruptured thoracic aortic aneurysm infected with listeria monocytogenes: A case report and a review of literature. Open Journal of Cardiovascular Surgery. 2013;**6**:1-7

[58] Anthuber M, Kemkes BM, Kreuzer E, Gokel M, Schuetz A, Kugler C, et al. Mediastinitis and mycotic aneurysm of the aorta after orthotopic heart transplantation. Texas Heart Institute Journal. 1991;**18**(3):186-193

Chapter 4

Human Immunodeficiency Virus Associated Large Artery Disease

Ruchika Meel and Ricardo Gonçalves

Abstract

Advances in human immunodeficiency virus (HIV) therapy with highly active antiretroviral agents has increased the longevity of patients afflicted with this disease. HIV vasculopathy is a unique disease entity presenting as aneurysms, dissections and vascular occlusion amongst others due to HIV related vasculitis. A few studies have investigated the pathogenesis of HIV related vasculopathy. This chapter provides a brief overview of aortic aneurysms in general. Further, the current understanding of the pathogenic mechanisms underlying HIV vasculopathy with an emphasis on inflammatory mediators, histology, clinical presentation and imaging are discussed. Finally, a summary regarding management of HIV associated large vessel disease is presented.

Keywords: HIV, vasculopathy, aneurysms

1. Introduction

Human immunodeficiency virus (HIV) is a global disease. According to global HIV and acquired immunodeficiency syndrome (AIDS) statistics in 2017, there were 36.9

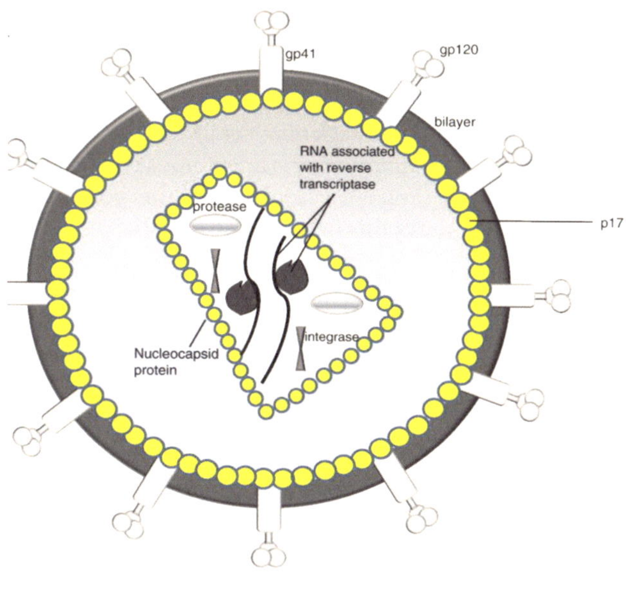

Figure 1.
Structure of the mature HIV virus. (Reproduced from Ref. [2]. Permission obtained from Michael S. Pepper).

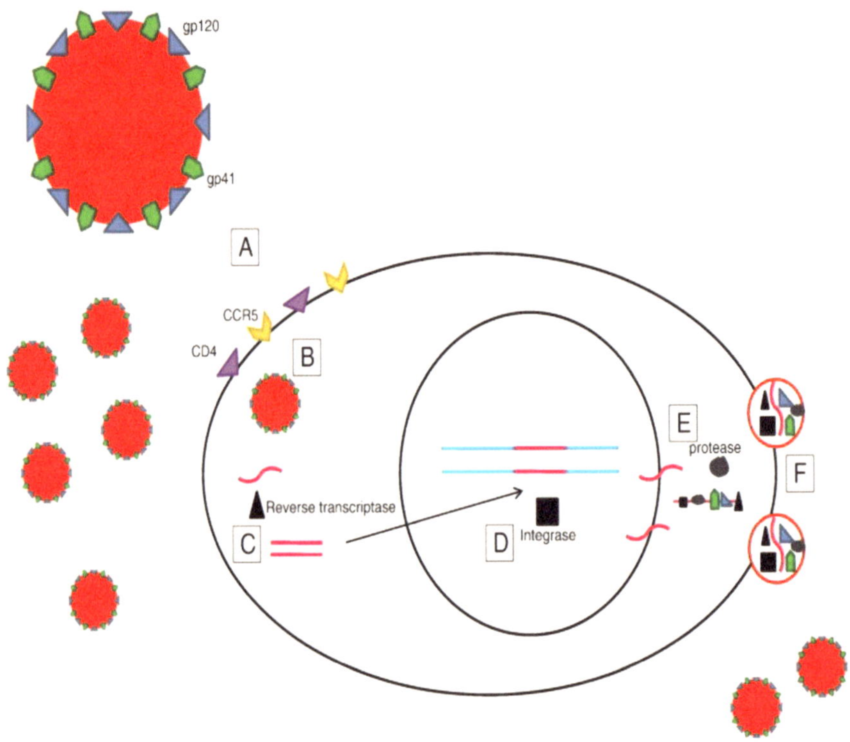

Figure 2.
Diagram illustrating HIV replication. (A) The virus glycoprotein receptors bind to host cell CD4 and a co-receptor CCR5. (B) Fusion of the virus with the host cell membrane results in viral uncoating and the release of the viral nucleocapsid into the cytoplasm. (C) The enzyme reverse transcriptase converts the single stranded RNA into double stranded DNA. (D) The viral DNA is transported to the host nucleus where it is integrated into the host's DNA. (E) Viral DNA is transcribed and translated using host cell machinery and then cleaved by viral protease into functional viral proteins. (F) Viral RNA and proteins assemble at the cell surface and bud off the cellular membrane. (Reproduced from Ref. [2]. Permission obtained from Michael S Pepper).

million [31.1–43.9 million] people living with HIV, of whom 35.1 million [29.6–41.7 million] adults. The majority of these individuals reside in the developing world [1].

HIV infection involves multiple systems including the cardiovascular system. A structure of the HIV virus and its replication in a cell are depicted in **Figures 1** and **2**. A large number of these patients present with vascular pathology [3, 4]. HIV afflicts the vascular system in multiple ways. Patients may present with a diverse array of aneurysms, occlusive disease, spontaneous arteriovenous fistulae and dissections. The precise pathogenesis of HIV related vasculitis remains poorly understood, a few recent studies have tried to address this issue [5].

In this chapter we will review the current knowledge pertaining to the important entity of HIV associated vasculopathy with an emphasis on effects of HIV on the aorta.

2. Definition and broad overview of aortic aneurysms

An aortic aneurysm is a dilation of a segment of the aortic wall, which may undergo further expansion and rupture [6]. It is defined as at least a 50% increase in diameter compared with the expected normal diameter of the vessel. They may occur in the ascending or the descending thoracic or abdominal aorta.

It may be fusiform or saccular in morphology [6]. A fusiform aneurysm is characterised by a uniform symmetric enlargement of the entire circumference of the aortic wall. A saccular aneurysm involves dilation of a localised portion of the aortic wall.

DOI: http://dx.doi.org/10.5772/intechopen.85956

These are true aneurysms as opposed to false aneurysms, as they involve all three layers of the aortic wall.

3. Aetiology

There are multiple aetiologies implicated in the pathogenesis of aortic aneurysms [6]. These include:

1. Degenerative or atherosclerotic diseases.

2. Genetic diseases, such as Marfan syndrome, Loeys-Dietz syndrome, Ehlers-Danlos syndrome, familial thoracic aortic aneurysms, bicuspid aortic valve disease, Turner syndrome and aortopathy associated with congenital heart disease.

3. Inflammatory diseases, such as Takayasu's disease and giant cell arteritis.

4. Infectious diseases, including bacterial infections (the most common organisms implicated are *Staphylococcus aureus*, *Salmonella* species, *Escherichia coli*, *Streptococcus* species, *Neisseria* species and gram-negative bacilli) and fungi. Recently, HIV has been implicated in the pathogenesis of aortic aneurysms. Infected aortic aneurysms have a high mortality.

4. Epidemiology

The true incidence and prevalence of aortic aneurysms is difficult to ascertain due to the silent nature of this disease [7]. In a computed chest tomography (CT) study the prevalence of asymptomatic thoracic ascending aneurysm was 0.16% [8]. In a different study the prevalence was noted to be 0.34% [9]. The incidence and prevalence of aneurysms tend to differ between studies due to different aortic dimension cut-offs. The majority of studies did not include aortas between 4 and 5 cm [7]. The annual incidence according to two studies was estimated to be in the range of 5.6 and 10.4 cases per 100,000 patient-years [10, 11]. Thoracic aneurysms are more common in men greater than 60 years of age [7].

Abdominal aortic aneurysm is predominantly a disease of men [12–15]. The incidence rises with age. In screening studies its prevalence is estimated at 4–8%. The incidence of new cases of abdominal aortic aneurysms in the western population is estimated at 0.4–0.67% [7].

The true incidence and prevalence of HIV associated aneurysms remains understudied. The incidence of symptomatic vasculitis in HIV-infected patients is reported to be 1% [16].

5. Pathogenesis of HIV associated vasculopathy

The pathogenesis of HIV associated vasculopathy is multifactorial (**Figure 3**) [5]. Three pathophysiological processes have been implicated:

- Inflammation and endothelial injury

- Smooth muscle cell proliferation and migration

- Molecular mimicry

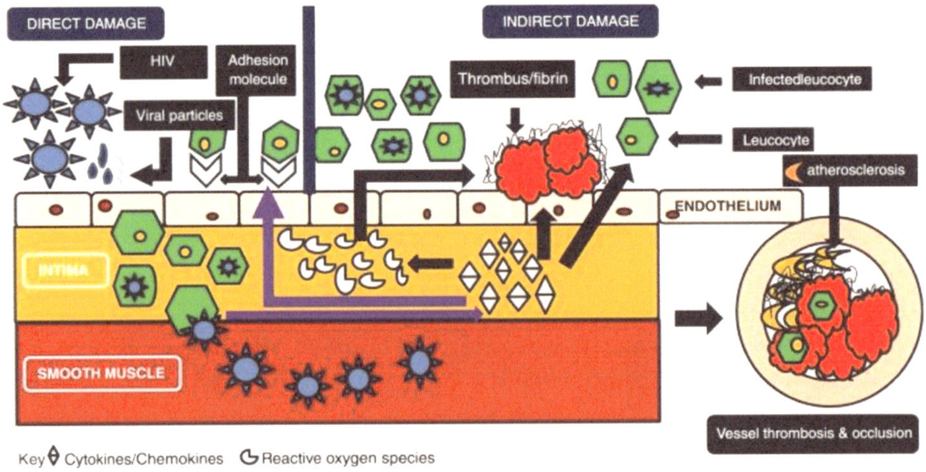

Figure 3.
Pathogenesis of HIV associated vasculopathy. (Reproduced from Ref. [5]. Permission obtained from B Pillay).

5.1 Inflammation and endothelial injury

Endothelial cell dysfunction as a result of increase in inflammatory mediators to viral proteins has been implicated in the pathogenesis of HIV related vasculitis [5]. The inflammatory mediators include interleukins 1, 6 and 8, and tumour necrosis factor-alpha. The aforementioned argument is supported by a study by Nieuwhof et al., in the setting of cerebral vasculitis, whereby, they found an increased CD25-positive receptor positive T-cells. HIV envelope surface glycoprotein 120 and a transactivator transcription protein that have been implicated in the stimulation of pro-inflammatory pathways in HIV related vasculitis.

Increased oxidative stress in HIV in animal studies has been proposed as an additional mechanism of endothelial dysfunction [17].

5.2 Smooth muscle cell proliferation and migration

Smooth muscle cells, an important component of the muscularis media, possess important surface receptors such as CD4, CCR5 and CXCR4 [5]. These receptors mediate the entry of HIV virus into the cell resulting in invasion and disruption of tunica media, and activation of tissue factor 2 with resultant stimulation of pro-coagulant pathways.

5.3 Molecular mimicry

It is theorised that the arterial wall possesses receptors known as matrix adhesion molecule-1 which may share ligands with similar deoxyribonucleic acid sequences to those present in the viral envelope glycoprotein, GP41 and GP120 [5]. This may result in an autoimmune response within the host and cell damage.

5.4 Other postulated mechanisms involved in the pathogenesis of HIV related vasculopathy

Direct invasion by HIV of vascular endothelium and toxicities related to highly active antiretroviral therapy (HAART) have been postulated as possible additional mechanisms resulting in endothelial injury [17].

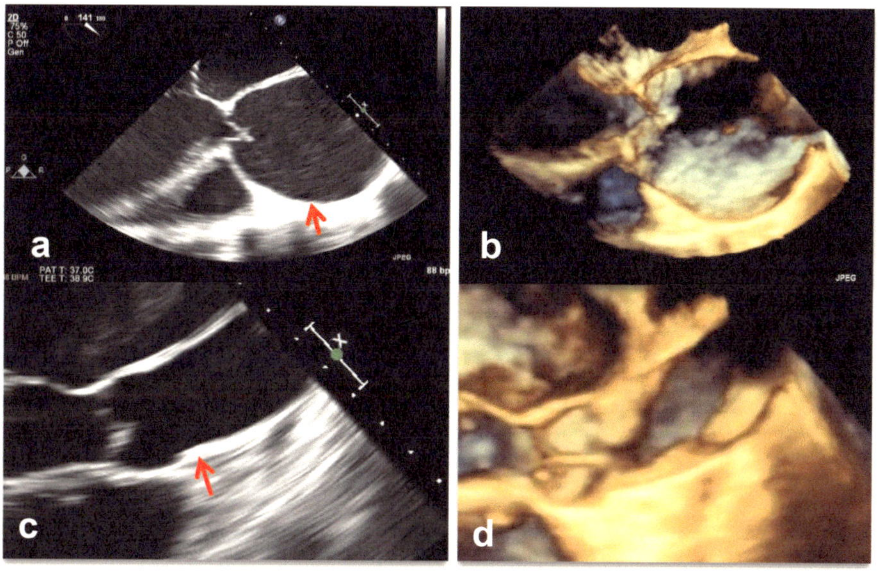

Figure 4.
Two and three dimensional long axis trans-oesophageal images of an enlarged ascending aorta in a patient with HIV associated aortopathy (arrow) (a, b) and a normal aorta in a control (arrow) (c, d).

5.5 HIV-associated aortopathy

HIV-associated aortopathy may present as aneurysmal disease of the ascending and the descending aorta (**Figure 4a–d**). Bacterial infections have been implicated in the pathogenesis of aortic aneurysms [5, 6]. A few case reports have reported the presence of *Salmonella*-related mycotic aneurysmal disease in HIV-positive patients. These aneurysms have been reported in immunosuppressed patients with advanced HIV disease [5].

5.6 Other forms of HIV related vasculopathy

HIV may affect femoral, carotid and popliteal arteries [5]. It may manifest as aneurysmal or occlusive disease as well as present as arterio-venous fistula and as arterial dissection. Since the advent of HAART, atherosclerotic disease is also a possible manifestation of HIV vasculopathy.

6. Histopathological features of HIV associated large vessel vasculopathy

Large vessel vasculopathy related to HIV is characterised by involvement of all three layers of the vessel wall [5]. There is infiltration of the vasa vasorum, periadventitial vessels and the adventitia by leucocytes. The media demonstrates fibrosis, muscle damage and elastin fragmentation. The intima also is characterised by disrupted internal elastic lamina and calcification.

Intracranial aneurysms due to HIV have been reported in children [5]. Overall histopathological studies have shown similar microscopic characteristics as previously described. Some studies, however, have shown distinct tissue characteristics in arteries of patients with intracranial aneurysms. These include variable absence of internal elastic lamina fragmentation, medial thickening with sub-intimal SMC deposition, presence of viral protein gp41 within the macrophages of the arterial wall, as well as identification of agents such as varicella zoster virus in the tissue.

7. Clinical features of HIV-associated large vessel vasculopathy

These patients will usually have stigmata of advanced HIV disease and presence of other opportunistic infections may confound the clinical picture.

The majority of patients with thoracic ascending aortic aneurysms and abdominal aortic aneurysms are asymptomatic [5, 18]. Symptoms usually result from large aneurysms and include chest or upper back pain, or with symptoms related to compression of nearby structures leading to nerve dysfunction, or compression of the artery resulting in limb ischemia or thromboembolism. The initial presentation may be aortic dissection or rupture and is associated with high mortality.

Abdominal aortic aneurysms may present with abdominal, back, or flank pain, thromboembolism or limb ischemia [19].

An enlarging aneurysm of the carotid artery may present with dysphagia, airway compromise, hoarse voice, cranial nerve involvement, cerebrovascular accident and even rupture [5].

Occlusive disease is another manifestation of HIV vasculopathy [5]. It usually involves young males below the age of 40 years. It afflicts lower limbs more commonly than upper limbs. Clinical presentation can be acute or chronic. Acute presentation involves arterial thrombosis or occlusion. Chronic disease may manifest as critical limb ischemia in the form of rest pain or gangrene in more than half of the patients.

8. Imaging in HIV associated vasculopathy

A basic chest radiograph is considered a reasonable initial test in a patient presenting with chest pain. It can exclude an alternative diagnosis and avoid unnecessary additional aortic imaging [18].

A transthoracic echocardiogram or transesophageal echocardiography are useful bedside tests to assess the presence of aortic enlargement and related complications such as aortic regurgitation, dissection and pericardial effusion.

Cardiac computed tomography and magnetic resonance angiography are the imaging modalities of choice and help determine the aortic size, branch vessel anatomy and presence of dissection (**Figure 5**) [18]. In patients with coexisting risk factors for coronary artery disease such as HIV, a cardiac CT is useful to exclude presence of coronary artery disease.

Digital subtraction arteriography provides higher resolution of lumen of the vessel and is better at evaluating branch vessel pathology [18].

The aortic measurements must be made at the aortic annulus, sinuses, sinotubular junction, ascending arch, and specific locations of the descending aorta as per the American society of echocardiography chamber quantification guidelines [20]. The aortic annulus is measured at peak systole whereas all other aortic dimensions are measured at end-diastole. Currently, a leading edge to leading edge method of measurement is recommended.

Large vessel disease has been studied with the aid of multiple imaging modalities. Arterial inflammation in patients with HIV has been demonstrated using ^{18}flourodeoxyglucose-positron emission tomography [21]. Inflammation is associated with an increased cardiovascular risk amongst HIV patients. Carotid intima-media thickness has been studied in these patients with the aid of ultrasound technology [22]. An increased carotid intima thickness is a marker of adverse cardiovascular disease.

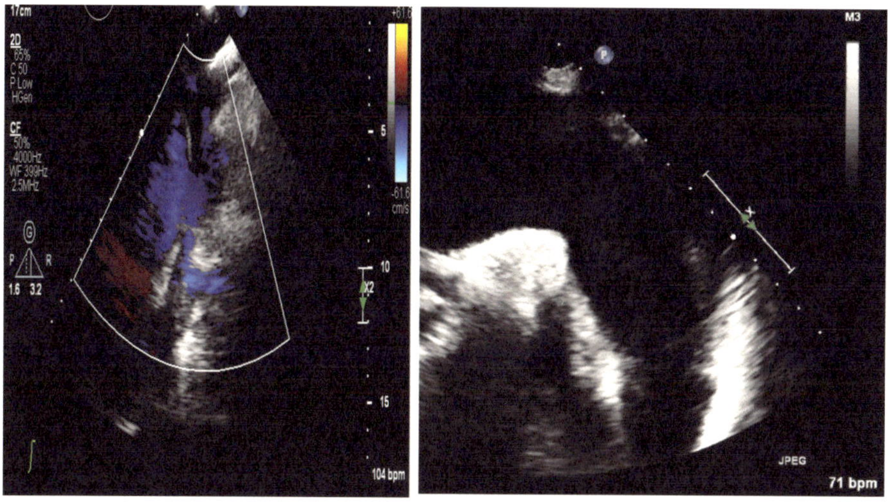

Figure 5.
Transthoracic echocardiographic suprasternal views of an enlarged aortic arch (right) and descending thoracic aorta dissection (left) in a patient with HIV.

The choice of imaging technique depends on the availability of resources and expertise to interpret the results of the test.

9. Management of patients with HIV vasculopathy

Currently all HIV patients with vascular disease must be managed according to standard guidelines [23]. Conservative management may be considered in a moribund severely immunosuppressed patient with multiple co-morbidities [5]. All patients must be on HAART therapy.

Data regarding management of ascending aortic aneurysm in patients with HIV is limited. Currently the standard guidelines on management of aortopathy are applied to these patients. Patients with ascending thoracic aortic aneurysms with symptoms due to aortic regurgitation, dissection and rupture should undergo emergent surgery as per the standard guidelines [23]. Those without symptoms but an enlarged ascending aorta greater than 55 mm are at high risk of rupture and dissection and therefore urgent surgery is recommended. Asymptomatic patients who display rapid growth of thoraco-abdominal aortic aneurysms, expansion ≥1 cm per year for aneurysms less than 50 mm in diameter, must undergo surgery [24]. Aortic diameter is an important risk factor for aneurysm rupture, dissection and mortality [6]. An ascending aorta diameter of 6.0 and 7.0 cm in the descending aorta is associated with increased risk of rupture.

In patients with multiple comorbidities and high risk for surgery conservative management with afterload reducing agents such as angiotensin converting enzyme inhibitors or angiotensin receptor antagonists, can be utilised to reduce the shear stress on the aorta and prevent further expansion and dissection [6, 25]. Beta blockers have been shown to decrease aortic stress and are recommended even in patients without systemic hypertension [6].

In centres where there is a lack of expertise in managing thoracic aortic disease, patients should be referred to an appropriate high volume centre in order to provide the best care and outcomes for such patients [25].

For descending aortic and peripheral artery aneurysms, depending on the site and location of the aneurysm patients can undergo surgical repair of the aneurysm with good success [5]. Patients that are unable to tolerate major surgery due to poor physiologic reserve can be offered endovascular repair. Data comparing endovascular repair versus surgery are limited in patients with HIV. Descending aortic aneurysms depending on the size and in absence of complications can be managed with medical therapy under close observation and follow-up [6].

The medical management of patients with HIV-related vasculopathy involves a combination of HAART, treatment of hyperlipidaemia and control of traditional risk factors associated with cardiovascular disease [5].

10. Prognosis and outcome

HIV patients with low CD4 counts, hyperglobulinemia, hypoalbuminemia and reversed CD4/CD8 ratios were reported have worse prognosis in a study by Van Marle et al. [26]. For peripheral large vessel surgery the perioperative mortality was reported to be between 9 and 10.6% in South Africa and 33% in Houston [5]. Major challenges related to wound healing and infection. Late graft sepsis rate of 10% has been reported with the use of prosthetic grafts. The follow-up in the aforementioned studies was poor and presents a major challenge in reporting long term outcomes. Further, the results may vary between patients on HAART compared to those without HAART. There are no studies pertaining to surgery in patients with ascending aortic aneurysms and descending thoracic aneurysms in the setting of HIV. No current studies address the natural history of HIV associated ascending or descending aortic aneurysms.

Conflict of interest

The authors have none to declare.

Funding

The first author was the recipient of the Carnegie Post-Doctoral Fellowship award.

Author details

Ruchika Meel[1]* and Ricardo Gonçalves[2]

1 Division of Cardiology, Chris Hani Baragwanath Academic Hospital and University of the Witwatersrand, Johannesburg, South Africa

2 Olivedale and Glynnwood Hospitals, Johannesburg, South Africa

*Address all correspondence to: ruchikameel@gmail.com

References

[1] Global HIV and AIDS statistics. https://www.hiv.gov/hiv-basics/overview/data-and-trends/global-statistics [Accessed: 24 November 2018]

[2] Barmania F, Pepper MS. C-C chemokine receptor type five (CCR5): An emerging target for the control of HIV infection. Applied & Translational Genomics. 2013;**2**:3-16

[3] Mulaudzi TV. HIV-associated vasculopathy. CME. 2009;**27**(7):320-322

[4] Robbs JV, Paruk N. Management of HIV vasculopathy: A South African experience. European Journal of Vascular and Endovascular Surgery. 2010;**39**(Suppl 1):S25-S31

[5] Pillay B, Ramdial PK, Naidoo DP. HIV-associated large-vessel vasculopathy: A review of the current and emerging clinicopathological spectrum in vascular surgical practice. Cardiovascular Journal of Africa. 2015;**26**(2):70

[6] Zipes DP, Libby P, Bonow RO, Mann DL, Tomaselli GF. Braunwald's Heart Disease: A Textbook of Cardiovascular Medicine. Elsevier Saunders; 2018

[7] Black JH III, Woo CL. Epidemiology, Risk Factors, Pathogenesis, and Natural History of Thoracic Aortic Aneurysm. Wolters Kluwer; 2017

[8] Itani Y, Watanabe S, Masuda Y, et al. Measurement of aortic diameters and detection of asymptomatic aortic aneurysms in a mass screening program using a mobile helical computed tomography unit. Heart Vessels. 2002;**16**:42

[9] Kälsch H, Lehmann N, Möhlenkamp S, et al. Body-surface adjusted aortic reference diameters for improved identification of patients with thoracic aortic aneurysms: Results from the population-based Heinz Nixdorf recall study. International Journal of Cardiology. 2013;**163**:72

[10] Bickerstaff LK, Pairolcro PC, Hollier LH, et al. Thoracic aortic aneurysms: A population-based study. Surgery. 1982;**92**:1103

[11] Clouse WD, Hallett JW Jr, Schaff HV, et al. Improved prognosis of thoracic aortic aneurysms: A population-based study. JAMA. 1998;**280**:1926

[12] Ashton HA, Buxton MJ, Day NE, et al. The Multicentre Aneurysm Screening Study (MASS) into the effect of abdominal aortic aneurysm screening on mortality in men: A randomised controlled trial. Lancet. 2002;**360**:1531

[13] Norman PE, Jamrozik K, Lawrence-Brown MM, et al. Population based randomised controlled trial on impact of screening on mortality from abdominal aortic aneurysm. BMJ. 2004;**329**:1259

[14] Lindholt JS, Juul S, Fasting H, Henneberg EW. Screening for abdominal aortic aneurysms: Single centre randomised controlled trial. BMJ. 2005;**330**:750

[15] Ashton HA, Gao L, Kim LG, et al. Fifteen-year follow-up of a randomized clinical trial of ultrasonographic screening for abdominal aortic aneurysms. The British Journal of Surgery. 2007;**94**:696

[16] Chang JM, Lameen H, Skinner GC. Multiple large vessel aneurysmal formation in HIV-infected patients. SA Journal of Radiology. 2017;**21**(2):a1186

[17] Baliga RS, Chaves AA, Jing L, Ayers LW, Bauer JA. AIDS-related vasculopathy: Evidence for oxidative and inflammatory pathways in murine

and human AIDS. American Journal of Physiology—Heart and Circulatory Physiology. 2005;**289**(4):H1373-H1380

[18] Woo YJ, Greene CL, Hoekstra J, Eidt JF. Clinical Manifestations and Diagnosis of Thoracic Aortic Aneurysm. Walthman, MA: UpToDate; 2014. Monografía en Internet

[19] Jim J, Thompson RW, Eidt JF. Clinical Features and Diagnosis of Abdominal Aortic Aneurysm. Wolters Kluwer; 2018

[20] Lang RM, Badano LP, Mor-Avi V, Afilalo J, Armstrong A, Ernande L, et al. Recommendations for cardiac chamber quantification by echocardiography in adults: An update from the American Society of Echocardiography and the European Association of Cardiovascular Imaging. European Heart Journal Cardiovascular Imaging. 2015;**16**(3):233-271

[21] Subramanian S, Tawakol A, Burdo TH, Abbara S, Wei J, Vijayakumar J, et al. Arterial inflammation in patients with HIV. Journal of the American Medical Association. 2012;**308**(4):379-386

[22] Stein JH, Currier JS, Hsue PY. Arterial disease in patients with human immunodeficiency virus infection: What has imaging taught us? JACC: Cardiovascular Imaging. 2014;7(5):515-525

[23] Authors/Task Force Members, Erbel R, Aboyans V, Boileau C, Bossone E, Bartolomeo RD, et al. 2014 ESC guidelines on the diagnosis and treatment of aortic diseases: Document covering acute and chronic aortic diseases of the thoracic and abdominal aorta of the adult. The Task Force for the Diagnosis and Treatment of Aortic Diseases of the European Society of Cardiology (ESC). European Heart Journal. 2014;**35**(41):2873-2926

[24] Lobato AC, Puech-Leão P. Predictive factors for rupture of thoracoabdominal aortic aneurysm. Journal of Vascular Surgery. 1998;**27**:446

[25] Woo J, Greene C, Connolly HM, Aldea FG, Verrier E. Management of Thoracic Aortic Aneurysm in Adults. Wolters Kluwer; 2017

[26] Van Marle J, Mistry PP, Botes K. HIV-occlusive vascular disease. South African Journal of Surgery. 2009;**47**(2):36-42

Chapter 5

A New Mouse Model of Aortic Aneurysm Induced by Deoxycorticosterone Acetate or Aldosterone in the Presence of High Salt

Ming C. Gong, Shu Liu and Zhenheng Guo

Abstract

The renin-angiotensin-aldosterone system (RAAS) is implicated in the etiologies of many cardiovascular diseases, including abdominal aortic aneurysm (AAA) and thoracic aortic aneurysm (TAA). In particular, the infusion of angiotensin II (Ang II) in hyperlipidemia mice to induce AAA and TAA has been extensively used in the field, suggesting a critical role of Ang II in aortic aneurysm. In contrast, whether aldosterone (Aldo), a downstream effector of Ang II, is involved in aortic aneurysm is unknown. Here, we describe a new mouse model of AAA and TAA induced by subcutaneous implantation of deoxycorticosterone acetate (DOCA) pellets or infusion of Aldo using osmotic pumps to 10-month-old C57BL/6 male mice in the presence of high salt. The DOCA- or Aldo-salt-induced aortic aneurysm is dependent upon mineralocorticoid receptor activation but independent of Ang II and hypertension and exhibits several unique features that mimic human aortic aneurysm. This review aims to discuss the common animal models of AAA, TAA, and aortic dissection currently studied in the world with the most focus on the DOCA- or Aldo-salt mouse model of aortic aneurysm.

Keywords: aortic aneurysm, angiotensin II, aldosterone, DOCA, high salt, animal model

1. Introduction

An aortic aneurysm is defined as a permanent localized dilation of the aorta with at least a 50% increase in diameter compared with a normal aortic diameter [1]. Aortic aneurysms can be classified according to location as thoracic aortic aneurysm (TAA) and abdominal aortic aneurysm (AAA). TAA occurs in all-age people without sexual dimorphism and is highly associated with hereditary conditions [2]. By contrast, AAA is typically associated with aging, male sex, smoking, atherosclerosis, and hypertension [3–5]. AAA is the most common form of aortic aneurysm [6], affecting 4–8% of men and 0.5–1.5% of women over the age of 60 and currently accounting for nearly 2% of all deaths in Western countries [2, 3, 7]. Aortic aneurysm is an asymptomatic condition that tends to progress over time with a high mortality rate (65–85%) if rupture occurs [8]. Unfortunately, repair through open or endovascular surgery is currently the only therapeutic option for aortic aneurysm; no drug has been approved for treatment of this devastating disease [3, 5]. One of the major barriers in the field is a lack of an animal model that fully resembles human aortic aneurysm.

Over the last few decades, a number of rodent models of AAA and TAA have been developed and have been increasingly utilized to be used in understanding the etiology of human AAA and TAA [2, 9–11]. Aortic aneurysm animal models can be classified into three groups [2, 9–11]: (1) genetically predisposed animal models (i.e., fibrillin-1 (FBN1) mutation (Marfan syndrome) mouse model [2, 12]), (2) chemical-induced animal models (i.e., Ang II infusion hyperlipidemia mouse model [9, 13]), and (3) physical or surgical animal models (i.e., decellularized aortic xenograft rat model [10, 14]). Among them, calcium chloride adventitial application model [15, 16], porcine pancreatic elastase (PPE) model [17, 18], and Ang II infusion hyperlipidemia mouse model [13, 19–23] are the commonest animal models currently studied in the world.

One of the fundamental pathological characteristics in human TAA and AAA is thoracic aortic dissection (TAD) and abdominal aortic dissection (AAD), both of which can lead to aneurysmal rupture with high mortality [1–7]. Many genetically predisposed animal models have TAD and AAD (i.e., fibrillin-1 mutation mouse model [2, 12]). Some of the chemical-induced animal models also have TAD and AAD (i.e., fibrillin-1 mutation and Ang II infusion hyperlipidemia mouse models [13, 19–23]). Recently, a new chemical-induced mouse model for more potently induction of TAD and AAD was developed by administration of β-aminopropionitrile monofumarate (BAPN) to mice to inhibit lysyl oxidase (LOX) and/or Ang II infusion [24, 25]. Kurihara et al. demonstrated that BAPN/Ang II induced TAD in 100% of FVB mice [24]. Ren et al. confirmed this finding and further demonstrated that BAPN/Ang II induced TAD and AAD in 75% of C57BL/6J mice, whereas BAPN alone induced TAD in 87% of C57BL/6J [25].

Although no single animal model fully reproduces the histological characteristics and natural history of the human aortic aneurysm, each of these animal models more or less recapitulate human aortic aneurysm and have significantly contributed to the current understanding of clinical management and treatment of patients with AAA and TAA [2, 9–11]. Several clinical trials have begun enrollment to examine whether angiotensin-converting enzyme (ACE) inhibitors or angiotensin receptor blockers (ARB) are effective in the treatment of human aortic aneurysm. However, the results from these clinical trials are inconsistent and disappointing: either effective [26], no effect [27], or, even worse [28], indicating that the current understanding about the etiologies of aortic aneurysm is limited and additional unknown signaling and mechanism may underlie aortic aneurysm and account for the failure of these clinical trials.

In sharp contrast to the well-established role of Ang II in aortic aneurysm [13, 19–23], little is known about the role of aldosterone (Aldo) in aortic aneurysm. Aldo is a steroid hormone primarily synthesized and released by the adrenal glands. Aldo is a downstream effect of Ang II and is well recognized for its critical role in renal sodium reabsorption and water retention and consequently extracellular volume and blood pressure [29, 30]. Accumulated data over the last decade, however, demonstrate that Aldo not only acts on the kidney but also targets many other organelles, including those in the cardiovascular system, where it is critically involved in diverse pathophysiological processes [31–33].

Several lines of clinical study implicate Aldo signaling in aortic aneurysm. First, individual case reports demonstrated that primary hyperaldosteronism is associated with aortic dissection [34–36]. Second, a retrospective study demonstrated that aldosteronism is associated with high morbidity and mortality from the early onset of hemorrhagic stroke and ruptured intracranial aneurysms [37]. Third, a few small studies have shown an association between obesity and increased levels of Aldo [38] and increased AAA [39]. Finally, perhaps also the most compellingly, an analysis of drug modulation of AAA development through 25 years of surveillance in 1269 patients demonstrated a strong association between mineralocorticoid receptor (MR; also known as Aldo receptor) blockers and slowed AAA progression [40]. However, whether Aldo causes aortic aneurysm is unknown.

By incidence, we discovered that administration of deoxycorticosterone acetate (DOCA) to 10-month-old C57BL/6 male mice caused substantial animal death in the presence of high salt due to aortic aneurysmal rupture. A subsequent serial of substantial studies demonstrated that activation of MR by either implantation of DOCA pellet or infusion of Aldo in 10-month-old C57BL/6 male mice was sufficient to induce AAA and TAA formation and aneurysmal rupture in the presence of high salt [41–43]. Recently, we published the detailed methodology on how to implant DOCA pellet or Aldo pumps to induce aortic aneurysm [44]. Here, we will focus on the significant novel finding of this new AAA mouse model, highlight its unique features that mimic human aortic aneurysm, and discuss its significance and potential impact on the current understanding, diagnosis, and treatment of human aortic aneurysm.

2. Development of a new mouse model of aortic aneurysm induced by DOCA- or Aldo-salt

2.1 Discovery of DOCA-salt mouse model of aortic aneurysm by accidence

In an independent pilot study using 10- to 12-month-old C57BL/6 male mice to investigate DOCA-salt-induced hypertension, we unexpectedly observed that many mice died from AAA rupture. We were intrigued by this observation since it raised the possibility that activation of the MR by DOCA can cause AAA in the presence of high salt. Given that administration of DOCA and salt to mice or rats have been used extensively as an experimental model of low-renin hypertension [45], it was surprising that DOCA-salt-induced AAA has not been reported in previous studies. While the exact reasons for this discrepancy are unclear, our results suggest that the age of mice (i.e., 10-month old *vs.* 10-week old) may be critical for DOCA and salt to induce AAA (see below).

2.2 Both DOCA and high salt are required to induce aortic aneurysm

To verify our pilot studies and define whether DOCA, salt, or both is critical for DOCA-salt-induced aortic aneurysm, 10-month-old C57BL/6 male mice received DOCA alone (subcutaneous implantation of DOCA pellets; 50 mg, 21-day release; Innovative Research of America, USA), salt alone (drinking water containing 0.9% NaCl plus 0.2% KCl), DOCA and salt, or no treatment (controls). We used C57BL/6 mice because C57BL/6 mice are more susceptible to chemical (i.e., BAPN/Ang II)-induced TAD, AAD, and aneurysmal rupture than other strains of mice (i.e., FVB mice) [24, 25]. We used 10-month-old rather than 10-week-old mice because we found that DOCA- or Aldo-salt-induced aortic aneurysm were aging dependent [41, 43]. We used male mice rather than female mice because DOCA- or Aldo-salt-induced aortic aneurysm has sex difference (unpublished data). All mice were euthanized 3 weeks after treatment.

We used three different approaches to quantify DOCA-salt-induced aortic aneurysm. First, the maximal intraluminal diameters of abdominal aortas were quantified in vivo by a high-resolution ultrasound imaging system (Vevo 2100, Visualsonics, Toronto, Canada). The results showed that both DOCA and salt but not DOCA or salt alone could potently induce abdominal aortic dilation relative to the control [41]. Second, the maximal external diameters of isolated abdominal and thoracic aortas were quantified ex vivo by Nikon SMZ800 Stereo Microscope with a digital camera and NIS-Elements software. Consistently with the ultrasound data, both DOCA and salt but not DOCA or salt alone significantly increased external diameters of abdominal and thoracic aortas relative to the control [41].

Third, we calculated the incidence of DOCA-sat-induced AAA, TAA, and aneurysmal rupture based on the definition that AAA or TAA has at least a 50% increase in diameter compared with the normal diameter of the aorta [1]. Of the 45 mice treated with DOCA-salt, 28 mice developed AAA (62%), 22 mice developed TAA (42%), and 8 mice died of aortic aneurysmal rupture (18%). In contrast, no AAA, TAA, or aortic aneurysmal rupture was observed in control, DOCA, or salt alone. Interestingly, AAA was only found in the suprarenal abdominal aorta, which is similar to that in the Ang II AAA mouse model [13], whereas TAA was mostly associated with AAA and was mostly observed in the descending thoracic aorta, indicating that TAA is likely derived from AAA.

2.3 Infusion of mice with Aldo can also induce aortic aneurysm in the presence of high salt

Since DOCA is a synthetic MR agonist, we wondered whether Aldo, a physiologic ligand of MR in our body, could induce aortic aneurysm in the presence of high salt. To define the concentration of Aldo that is sufficient to induce aortic aneurysm in the presence of high salt, 10-month-old C57BL/6 male mice were infused with three different doses of Aldo (200, 500, and 700 μg/kg/day) for 4 weeks. Aldo was delivered to mice via subcutaneous implantation of osmotic minipump (Alzet model 2004; DURECT, USA) containing Aldo solubilized in 50% DMSO. All groups of mice were treated for 4 weeks.

Infusion of mice with all three doses of Aldo was very similar to implantation of mice with DOCA pellets and markedly increased maximal intraluminal and external diameters of suprarenal abdominal aortas compared to the control mice (without treatment). Similarly, infusion of mice with all three doses of Aldo is also similar to implantation of mice with DOCA pellets and potently induced AAA (over 58%), TAA (over 42%), and aneurysmal rupture (over 25%) compared to the control mice. These data demonstrated that the infusion of mice with 200 μg/kg/day Aldo is sufficient to induce AAA in the presence of high salt.

We measured the plasma Aldo concentrations by a commercial EIA kit (Enzo Life Science, USA) 4 weeks after Aldo and salt administration. We found that plasma Aldo concentrations were elevated in a dose-dependent manner. Of note, infusions of mice with 200 μg/kg/day Aldo resulted in plasma Aldo concentrations to ~10 nM, which could be seen in some human diseases such as congestive heart failure and primary aldosteronism [31, 46, 47]. These results indicate that the Aldo-salt AAA mouse model is a physiopathological model that mimics human diseases rather than a pharmacological model that would cause concerns due to the use of high doses of reagent.

2.4 DOCA-salt-induced aortic aneurysm is independent of Ang II

Although systematic plasma renin and Ang II concentrations are suppressed in animals administered with DOCA and salt [45], local aortic Ang II concentration can be increased due to activation of vascular RAAS, which was thought to be of pathophysiological relevance to the development of atherosclerosis [48]. Moreover, there is a synergistic interaction between Ang II and Aldo in VSMCs [49, 50]. Therefore, it is interesting to investigate whether DOCA-salt-induced aortic aneurysm is dependent upon Ang II. To address this important question, 10-month-old C57BL/6 male mice were treated with either an ACE inhibitor (enalapril) or an ARB (losartan) before (1 week) and after (4 weeks) DOCA-salt administration. As expected, enalapril or losartan effectively decreased blood pressure, but enalapril or losartan had little effect on the DOCA-salt-induced aortic dilation, aortic aneurysm formation, and aneurysmal rupture [41]. These results demonstrate that the DOCA-salt-induced aortic aneurysm is independent of Ang II thus provide an alternative mouse model of aortic aneurysm for investigators in the field who need an Ang II-independent mouse model to verify their key findings.

2.5 Activation of MR is a prerequisite for DOCA- or Aldo-salt to induce aortic aneurysm

To define the role of MR in DOCA- or Aldo-salt-induced aortic aneurysm, we treated 10-month-old C57BL/6 male mice with an MR antagonist eplerenone 1 week before and 4 weeks after Aldo-salt administration [41]. Eplerenone (Pfizer, USA) was delivered by feeding mice with custom diets (chow supplemented with eplerenone at 2.5 mg/g, Research Diets, Inc., USA). In contrast to the minimal effect of blocking Ang II with enalapril or losartan, treatment of mice with eplerenone completely abolished Aldo-salt-induced aortic dilation, AAA formation, and aortic aneurysmal rupture [41]. A similar but less potent effect on DOCA-salt-induced AAA was also found in mice treated with spironolactone [41]. These results suggest that activation of MR by DOCA or Aldo is a prerequisite for DOCA- or Aldo-salt to induce aortic aneurysm.

2.6 DOCA-salt induces aortic aneurysm independent of increased blood pressure

Administration of DOCA and salt to mice or rats has been used in the field to induce hypertension [45]. Hypertension is recognized as a potential risk factor for aortic aneurysm [3–5]. Thus, it is important to determine whether hypertension contributes to DOCA-salt-induced aortic aneurysm. Blood pressure was measured using a noninvasive tail-cuff system (Coda 6; Kent Scientific Corp., USA). As expected, administration of DOCA or Aldo plus salt to 10-month-old male mice increased both blood pressure and external diameters of the abdominal aorta [41, 43]. However, there was no correlation between blood pressure increase and external diameters of abdominal aorta after DOCA-salt treatment. Similarly, there was also no difference in blood pressure between the mice with aortic aneurysm and the mice without aortic aneurysm. Moreover, treatment of mice with ACE inhibitor enalapril or ARB losartan effectively decreased blood pressure, but both enalapril and losartan had little effect on DOCA-salt-induced aortic aneurysm. Thus, we concluded that DOCA-salt induces aortic aneurysm independent of increased blood pressure. This conclusion is consistent with that in the Ang II infusion AAA mouse model [19].

2.7 Vascular pathology of DOCA- or Aldo-salt induced aortic aneurysms

Human aortic aneurysm is characterized by elastin and collagen degradation, matrix metalloproteinase (MMP), upregulation, inflammatory cell infiltration, vascular smooth muscle cell degeneration, and oxidative stress [51]. To investigate whether DOCA- or Aldo-salt-induced aortic aneurysms have these pathologic features, paraffin-embedded aortic cross-sections were subjected to Elastic-Van Gieson staining of elastin. Interestingly, elastin degradation was only observed in AAA induced by DOCA- or Aldo-salt [41, 43]. Immunocytochemistry studies revealed that MMP2, MMP9, F4/80 (macrophages), Ly6B2 (neutrophils), caldesmon (smooth muscle cells), terminal deoxynucleotidyl transferase dUTP nick end labeling (TUNEL; apoptosis), and dihydroethidium (DHE; oxidative stress) were increased in aortas with AAA compared with that in control aortas [41, 43].

In agreement with these immunocytochemical studies, we determined mRNA expression of several inflammatory genes, including vascular cell adhesion molecule 1 (Vcam-1), chemokine (C-C motif) ligand 2 (Ccl2, also known as MCP-1), tumor necrosis factor (Tnf), and Ncf1 (also known as $p47^{phox}$) in both abdominal and thoracic aortas from mice-administrated DOCA-salt or control mice. We found that Vcam-1, Ccl2, Ncf1, and Tnf were all markedly upregulated in thoracic aortas from mice-administrated DOCA-salt compared to control mice. Interestingly, Vcam-1, Ccl2, and Ncf1, but not Tnf, were also significantly upregulated by DOCA-salt in abdominal aorta from mice-administrated DOCA-salt compared to control mice [41, 43].

2.8 Unique features of the DOCA- or Aldo-salt mouse model of aortic aneurysm

The DOCA- or Aldo-salt mouse model exhibited several unique features that may be relevant to the human aortic aneurysm. First, DOCA- or Aldo-salt-induced aortic aneurysm required to use 10-month-old mice [41, 43] rather than 10-week-old mice (mostly used by the Ang II AAA mouse model [13, 19–23] and other chemical-induced mouse modes [17, 18, 24, 25]). Given the fact that human AAA occurs in old peoples [2, 3, 7], the DOCA- or Aldo-salt mouse model of aortic aneurysm may more resemble human AAA than other chemical-induced aortic aneurysms in this regard. Second, DOCA- or Aldo-salt-induced aortic aneurysm used wild-type C57BL/6 mice [41, 43] rather than hyperlipidemia mice (i.e., apolipoprotein E-deficient ($ApoE^{-/-}$) used by Ang II infusion mouse models [13, 19–23]), thus avoiding the potential confounding effects of hyperlipidemia on aortic aneurysm. Third, using Aldo, a physiological agonist of MR, rather than chemicals (i.e., calcium chloride or pancreatic elastase) to induce aortic aneurysm, highlights its potential role in the etiology of aortic aneurysm. Moreover, the plasma concentration of Aldo in mice infused with Aldo [41] could be seen in human congestive heart failure and primary aldosteronism [31, 46, 47], suggesting that the Aldo-salt AAA mouse model is a pathological model rather than a pharmacological model that would cause concerns due to the use of high doses of reagent. Finally, high salt intake was required for DOCA to induce aortic aneurysm [41], indicating that high salt intake may be a new risk factor for the development of human AAA.

2.9 Significance and potential impact of the DOCA- or Aldo-salt mouse model of aortic aneurysm

We described a new mouse model of aortic aneurysm induced by administration of MR agonist DOCA or Aldo plus high salt to 10-month-old male mice and provided compelling preclinical evidence that reveals a previously unrecognized, but potentially significant, role of Aldo, MR, and high salt in the pathogenesis of AAA. It is worth pointing out that this new mouse model of aortic aneurysm could be used as a platform to study intervention including medication (i.e., we have tested the effect of ACE inhibitor (enalapril), ARB (losartan), and MR antagonist (eplerenone and spironolactone) [41]). It is also worth pointing out at least three significance and potential impact of the DOCA- or Aldo-salt mouse model of aortic aneurysm on the current basic research and clinical practice on the etiology, clinic diagnosis, evaluation, and treatment of AAA.

First, in agreement with the pivotal role of Aldo in cardiovascular diseases (i.e., hypertension and heart failure) [31, 32, 46], our studies highlight a potentially important but previously unrecognized role of Aldo in the etiology of human aortic aneurysm. Our studies suggest that increased plasma concentration of Aldo may be a new risk factor for human aortic aneurysm or may serve as a new plasma biomarker for evaluation of aortic aneurysm progression.

Second, it is well recognized that unfavorably excessive dietary sodium intakes remain prevalent around the world and are associated with an increased risk for cardiovascular diseases including hypertension, stroke, coronary heart disease, heart failure, and renal disease [52–54]. However, it is unknown that excessive dietary sodium intake may also be detrimental to the aorta with respect to aortic aneurysm. Our finding that excessive dietary sodium intake was essential for MR agonist to induce aortic aneurysm in mice suggests that excessive dietary sodium intakes may also be implicated in the etiology of human aortic aneurysm. In agreement with our findings, it was recently reported that high salt intake was associated with an increased prevalence of AAA in older men [55]. Moreover, our findings indicate that lifestyle change such as reduction of dietary sodium intakes may be effective to prevent old people from the development and progression of aortic aneurysm.

Third, given the fact that currently there is no approved drug for treatment of AAA, our studies suggest that spironolactone and eplerenone, two clinically approved drugs that have been used for the treatment of human heart failure and essential hypertension [56], may also be effective in the treatment of human aortic aneurysm. Recently, a proof-of-concept randomized controlled clinical trial has been initiated based on our findings and is currently going on in Australia, which aims to test the effect of eplerenone on the progression of AAA (https://clinicaltrials.gov/ct2/show/study/NCT02345590).

3. Conclusions

1. Subcutaneous implantation of MR agonist DOCA pellets to 10-month-old C57BL/6 male mice can potently induce aortic aneurysm formation and rupture in the presence of high salt. Both DOCA and salt, but not DOCA or salt alone, are required to induce aortic aneurysm formation and rupture in mice.

2. Infusion of 10-month-old C57BL/6 male mice by subcutaneous implantation of osmotic pumps to release Aldo to a pathological level can also induce aortic aneurysm formation and rupture, suggesting that increased plasma concentration of Aldo may be implicated in the etiology of human aortic aneurysm.

3. DOCA- or Aldo-salt-induced AAA mimics human AAA with respect to elastin degradation, MMP activation, inflammatory cell infiltration, smooth muscle cell degeneration, and oxidative stress.

4. Treatment of mice with ACE inhibitor enalapril or an ARB losartan has little effect on DOCA-salt-induced aortic aneurysm, suggesting that DOCA-salt-induced aortic aneurysm is independent of Ang II.

5. Treatment of mice with MR antagonist spironolactone and eplerenone effectively abolishes or diminishes DOCa- or Aldo-salt-induced aortic aneurysm,

suggesting that activation of MR is a prerequisite for DOCA- or Aldo-salt to induce aortic aneurysm, and more importantly, spironolactone and eplerenone, two clinically approved drugs, may also be effective for the treatment of some aortic aneurysm.

6. There is no correlation between blood pressure and aortic dilation or AAA formation in the DOCA- or Aldo-salt mouse model of aortic aneurysm, suggesting that DOCA-salt induces AAA independent of increased blood pressure.

Acknowledgements

This work was supported by the US National Institutes of Health (NIH) Grants HL125228 and HL106843 and HL142973 (to M.C.G. and Z.G.), the US Department of Veteran Affairs I01BX002141 (to Z.G.), and the Institutional Development Award (IDeA) from the US National Institute of General Medical Sciences of NIH, under grant number P30 GM127211.

Conflict of interest

The authors have no potential conflicts of interest with respect to the research, authorship, and publication of this article.

Author details

Ming C. Gong[1,3], Shu Liu[1,3,4] and Zhenheng Guo[2,3,4]*

1 Department of Physiology, Lexington, Kentucky, USA

2 Department of Pharmacology and Nutritional Science, Lexington, Kentucky, USA

3 Saha Cardiovascular Research Center, University of Kentucky, Lexington, Kentucky, USA

4 Research and Development, Lexington Veterans Affairs Medical Center, Lexington, Kentucky, USA

*Address all correspondence to: zguo2@uky.edu

References

[1] Hiratzka LF et al. 2010 ACCF/AHA/AATS/ACR/ASA/SCA/SCAI/SIR/STS/SVM Guidelines for the diagnosis and management of patients with thoracic aortic disease. A Report of the American College of Cardiology Foundation/American Heart Association Task Force on Practice Guidelines, American Association for Thoracic Surgery, American College of Radiology , American Stroke Association, Society of Cardiovascular Anesthesiologists, Society for Cardiovascular Angiography and Interventions, Society of Interventional Radiology, Society of Thoracic Surgeons, and Society for Vascular Medicine. Journal of the American College of Cardiology. 2010;**55**(14):e27-e129

[2] Lindsay ME, Dietz HC. Lessons on the pathogenesis of aneurysm from heritable conditions. Nature. 2011;**473**(7347):308-316

[3] Golledge J et al. Abdominal aortic aneurysm: Pathogenesis and implications for management. Arteriosclerosis, Thrombosis, and Vascular Biology. 2006;**26**(12):2605-2613

[4] Fleming C et al. Screening for abdominal aortic aneurysm: A best-evidence systematic review for the U.S. Preventive Services Task Force. Annals of Internal Medicine. 2005;**142**(3):203-211

[5] Baxter BT, Terrin MC, Dalman RL. Medical management of small abdominal aortic aneurysms. Circulation. 2008;**117**(14):1883-1889

[6] Isselbacher EM. Thoracic and abdominal aortic aneurysms. Circulation. 2005;**111**(6):816-828

[7] Weintraub NL. Understanding abdominal aortic aneurysm. The New England Journal of Medicine. 2009;**361**(11):1114-1116

[8] Forsdahl SH et al. Risk factors for abdominal aortic aneurysms: A 7-year prospective study: The Tromso Study, 1994-2001. Circulation. 2009;**119**(16):2202-2208

[9] Daugherty A, Cassis LA. Mouse models of abdominal aortic aneurysms. Arteriosclerosis, Thrombosis, and Vascular Biology. 2004;**24**(3):429-434

[10] Senemaud J et al. Translational relevance and recent advances of animal models of abdominal aortic aneurysm. Arteriosclerosis, Thrombosis, and Vascular Biology. 2017;**37**(3):401-410

[11] Tsui JC. Experimental models of abdominal aortic aneurysms. Open Cardiovascular Medicine Journal. 2010;**4**:221-230

[12] Attenhofer Jost CH et al. Medical treatment of aortic aneurysms in Marfan syndrome and other heritable conditions. Current Cardiology Reviews. 2014;**10**(2):161-171

[13] Daugherty A, Manning MW, Cassis LA. Angiotensin II promotes atherosclerotic lesions and aneurysms in apolipoprotein E-deficient mice. The Journal of Clinical Investigation. 2000;**105**(11):1605-1612

[14] Allaire E et al. Cell-free arterial grafts: Morphologic characteristics of aortic isografts, allografts, and xenografts in rats. Journal of Vascular Surgery. 1994;**19**(3):446-456

[15] Gertz SD, Kurgan A, Eisenberg D. Aneurysm of the rabbit common carotid artery induced by periarterial application of calcium chloride in vivo. The Journal of Clinical Investigation. 1988;**81**(3):649-656

[16] Lee JK et al. Experimental abdominal aortic aneurysms in mice lacking expression of inducible nitric oxide synthase. Arteriosclerosis,

Thrombosis, and Vascular Biology. 2001;**21**(9):1393-1401

[17] Anidjar S et al. Elastase-induced experimental aneurysms in rats. Circulation. 1990;**82**(3):973-981

[18] Pyo R et al. Targeted gene disruption of matrix metalloproteinase-9 (gelatinase B) suppresses development of experimental abdominal aortic aneurysms. The Journal of Clinical Investigation. 2000;**105**(11):1641-1649

[19] Cassis LA et al. ANG II infusion promotes abdominal aortic aneurysms independent of increased blood pressure in hypercholesterolemic mice. American Journal of Physiology. Heart and Circulatory Physiology. 2009;**296**(5):H1660-H1665

[20] Cassis LA et al. Aldosterone does not mediate angiotensin II-induced atherosclerosis and abdominal aortic aneurysms. British Journal of Pharmacology. 2005;**144**(3):443-448

[21] Rateri DL et al. Endothelial cell-specific deficiency of Ang II type 1a receptors attenuates Ang II-induced ascending aortic aneurysms in LDL receptor−/− mice. Circulation Research. 2011;**108**(5):574-581

[22] Zhang X et al. Transient exposure of neonatal female mice to testosterone abrogates the sexual dimorphism of abdominal aortic aneurysms. Circulation Research. 2012;**110**(11):e73-e85

[23] Thomas M et al. Deletion of p47phox attenuates angiotensin II-induced abdominal aortic aneurysm formation in apolipoprotein E-deficient mice. Circulation. 2006;**114**(5):404-413

[24] Kurihara T et al. Neutrophil-derived matrix metalloproteinase 9 triggers acute aortic dissection. Circulation. 2012;**126**(25):3070-3080

[25] Ren W et al. beta-Aminopropionitrile monofumarate induces thoracic aortic dissection in C57BL/6 mice. Scientific Reports. 2016;**6**:28149

[26] Kristensen KE et al. Angiotensin-converting enzyme inhibitors and angiotensin II receptor blockers in patients with abdominal aortic aneurysms: Nation-wide cohort study. Arteriosclerosis, Thrombosis, and Vascular Biology. 2015;**35**(3):733-740

[27] Kiru G et al. An evaluation of the effect of an angiotensin-converting enzyme inhibitor on the growth rate of small abdominal aortic aneurysms: a randomised placebo-controlled trial (AARDVARK). Health Technology Assessment. 2016;**20**(59):1-180

[28] Sweeting MJ et al. Use of angiotensin converting enzyme inhibitors is associated with increased growth rate of abdominal aortic aneurysms. Journal of Vascular Surgery: Official Publication, the Society for Vascular Surgery [and] International Society for Cardiovascular Surgery, North American Chapter. 2010;**52**(1):1-4

[29] Skott O et al. Rapid actions of aldosterone in vascular health and disease—Friend or foe? Pharmacology & Therapeutics. 2006;**111**(2):495-507

[30] Gilbert KC, Brown NJ. Aldosterone and inflammation. Current Opinion in Endocrinology, Diabetes, and Obesity. 2010;**17**(3):199-204

[31] Funder JW, Reincke M. Aldosterone: A cardiovascular risk factor? Biochimica et Biophysica Acta. 2010;**1802**(12):1188-1192

[32] Brown NJ. Eplerenone: Cardiovascular protection. Circulation. 2003;**107**(19):2512-2518

[33] McCurley A, Jaffe IZ. Mineralocorticoid receptors in

vascular function and disease. Molecular and Cellular Endocrinology. 2012;**350**(2):256-265

[34] Ahmed SH et al. Is primary hyperaldosteronism a risk factor for aortic dissection? Cardiology. 2007;**108**(1):48-50

[35] Hirai H et al. Simultaneous surgery for chronic aortic dissection and adrenal adenoma with primary aldosteronism. General Thoracic and Cardiovascular Surgery. 2010;**58**(5):235-237, discussion 238

[36] Podgorski M et al. Aortic dissection—A rare complication of primary aldosteronism—A case report. Kardiologia Polska. 2011;**69**(2):156-158, discussion 159

[37] Litchfield WR et al. Intracranial aneurysm and hemorrhagic stroke in glucocorticoid-remediable aldosteronism. Hypertension. 1998;**31** (1 Pt 2):445-450

[38] Flynn C. Increased aldosterone: Mechanism of hypertension in obesity. Seminars in Nephrology. 2014;**34**(3):340-348

[39] Cronin O, Walker PJ, Golledge J. The association of obesity with abdominal aortic aneurysm presence and growth. Atherosclerosis. 2013;**226**(2):321-327

[40] Thompson A et al. An analysis of drug modulation of abdominal aortic aneurysm growth through 25 years of surveillance. Journal of Vascular Surgery: Official Publication, the Society for Vascular Surgery [and] International Society for Cardiovascular Surgery, North American Chapter. 2010;**52**(1):55-61, e2

[41] Liu S et al. Mineralocorticoid receptor agonists induce mouse aortic aneurysm formation and rupture in the presence of high salt. Arteriosclerosis, Thrombosis, and Vascular Biology. 2013;**33**(7):1568-1579

[42] Golledge J. Is there a new target in the renin-angiotensin system for aortic aneurysm therapy? Arteriosclerosis, Thrombosis, and Vascular Biology. 2013;**33**(7):1456-1457

[43] Lutshumba J et al. Deletion of BMAL1 in smooth muscle cells protects mice from abdominal aortic aneurysms. Arteriosclerosis, Thrombosis, and Vascular Biology. 2018;**38**(5):1063-1075

[44] Liu S, Gong MC, Guo Z. A new mouse model for introduction of aortic aneurysm by implantation of deoxycorticosterone acetate pellets or aldosterone infusion in the presence of high salt. Methods in Molecular Biology. 2017;**1614**:155-163

[45] Schenk J, McNeill JH. The pathogenesis of DOCA-salt hypertension. Journal of Pharmacological and Toxicological Methods. 1992;**27**(3):161-170

[46] Weber KT. Aldosterone in congestive heart failure. The New England Journal of Medicine. 2001;**345**(23):1689-1697

[47] Rousseau MF et al. Beneficial neurohormonal profile of spironolactone in severe congestive heart failure: Results from the RALES neurohormonal substudy. Journal of the American College of Cardiology. 2002;**40**(9):1596-1601

[48] Weiss D, Taylor WR. Deoxycorticosterone acetate salt hypertension in apolipoprotein E−/− mice results in accelerated atherosclerosis: The role of angiotensin II. Hypertension. 2008;**51**(2):218-224

[49] Min LJ et al. Aldosterone and angiotensin II synergistically induce mitogenic response in vascular smooth muscle cells. Circulation Research. 2005;**97**(5):434-442

[50] Montezano AC et al. Aldosterone and angiotensin II synergistically

stimulate migration in vascular smooth muscle cells through c-Src-regulated redox-sensitive RhoA pathways. Arteriosclerosis, Thrombosis, and Vascular Biology. 2008;**28**(8):1511-1518

[51] Curci JA. Digging in the "soil" of the aorta to understand the growth of abdominal aortic aneurysms. Vascular. 2009;**17**(Suppl 1):S21-S29

[52] Powles J et al. Global, regional and national sodium intakes in 1990 and 2010: A systematic analysis of 24 h urinary sodium excretion and dietary surveys worldwide. BMJ Open. 2013;**3**(12):e003733

[53] Whelton PK et al. Sodium, blood pressure, and cardiovascular disease: Further evidence supporting the American Heart Association sodium reduction recommendations. Circulation. 2012;**126**(24):2880-2889

[54] Appel LJ et al. The importance of population-wide sodium reduction as a means to prevent cardiovascular disease and stroke: A call to action from the American Heart Association. Circulation. 2011;**123**(10):1138-1143

[55] Golledge J et al. Reported amount of salt added to food is associated with increased all-cause and cancer-related mortality in older men in a prospective Cohort study. The Journal of Nutrition, Health & Aging. 2015;**19**(8):805-811

[56] Maron BA, Leopold JA. Aldosterone receptor antagonists: Effective but often forgotten. Circulation. 2010;**121**(7):934-939

Chapter 6

Extensive Repair in Type A Aortic Dissection: To Save the Patient or to Ensure a Durable Repair?

Benoit Cosset, Sarah Abdellaoui, Hugo Huvelle, Amine Fikani and Fadi Farhat

Abstract

Type A aortic dissection (TAAD) is a serious condition requiring emergency surgical management. The main objective of the treatment is the patient survival. Thus, the surgeon has to perform a well-mastered surgical technique without extending the operative time and emphasizing operative risk. Nevertheless, patients with history of TAAD present long-term complications on the aorta, mainly aneurysmal evolution and dissection recurrence. In order to decrease the long-term excess mortality of this population, it is necessary to respect some rules during the surgery. Concerning the proximal segment of the ascending aorta, the aortic root has to be replaced by a composite graft (Bentall technique) or a valve sparing inclusion (David technique) when the dissection reaches the sinuses of Valsalva or when aortic valve regurgitation is observed. Concerning the distal segment of the ascending aorta, the distal anastomosis has to be performed without aortic clamping. Concerning the descending thoracic aorta, hybrid surgery should be performed on patients with malperfusion syndrome and patients with high risk factors for aneurysmal evolution.

Keywords: type A aortic dissection, aneurysm formation, extensive repair, aortic valve sparing, frozen elephant trunk

1. Introduction

Type A aortic dissection (TAAD) represents a double challenge: a short-term challenge with a 30-day mortality around 25% [1] and a long-term challenge with an excess of morbidity and mortality for this population [2]. Concerning the short-term evolution, the intrahospital mortality is mainly influenced by patient history and preoperative complications [2]. Concerning the long-term evolution, the excess of morbidity and mortality seems correlated to two main complications: complications of hypertension such as strokes and ischemic heart disease and complications of aneurysmal evolution of the descending aorta such as aortic rupture and reoperations [3]. Thus, the main challenge of the surgical management of the TAAD is to strike a balance between keeping an early mortality rate as low as possible and preventing long-term morbidity.

2. Save the patient

2.1 Short-term mortality: statistics and causes

Type A aortic dissection (TAAD) is a serious pathology with high short-term mortality rates. Indeed, series find a 50% mortality at 48 hours for nonoperated patients and an intrahospital mortality between 20 and 30% for operated patients [1].

This high mortality rate is due to the great number of serious complications associated to the TAAD. The main mortality cause in the TAAD is acute aortic rupture [1]. Concerning the cardiac complications, we observe an aortic regurgitation in 40–75% [4, 5], a cardiac tamponade in 20%, and a myocardial infarction in 10–15%. These complications lead to congestive heart failure in 10% of cases. The other complications are neurological such as spinal ischemia, stroke and coma, mesenteric ischemia, and renal failure.

The analysis of short-term mortality shows that the characteristics of the patient (age, history of aortic valve replacement) and the preoperative complications of the TAAD (migrating chest pain, preoperative limb ischemia, hypotension, shock, cardiac tamponade) have more impact on the early survival than the type of surgical management [2]. These results demonstrate that even with optimal medical and surgical management, TAAD will remain a serious pathology with high mortality rate. These short-term mortality risk factors distinguish the patients in two categories at the time of the surgery: stable patients and unstable patients. Patients are defined as unstable in case of cardiac tamponade, myocardial ischemia, congestive heart failure, shock, cerebrovascular accident, coma, mesenteric ischemia, and acute renal failure. The latter having short-term mortality rate twice as high as stable patients (31.4 versus 16.7%) [2]. This distinction is important for the choice of the surgical technique, which should depend in part upon the stability of the patient at the time of the surgery.

Management of patients with neurological complications at the onset of the dissection is still debated. To assess this issue, Tsukube presented the results of patients with coma on arrival [6]. They decided to operate immediately when coma was inferior to 5 hours. The surgical technique was a central repair performed under deep hypothermia with anterograde cerebral perfusion. For this group, intrahospital mortality was equal to 14%. Concerning the other patients, they were treated initially medically and in a second time surgically. Intrahospital mortality was equal to 67%. In terms of severity, the national institute of health stroke scale decreased significantly after the surgery in the immediate group. These results, confirmed by other series [7], show that coma, if managed immediately, should not be an operative contraindication.

Concerning the management of acute neurological deficit, Estrera showed that this complication, when managed surgically by central repair, was associated with an acceptable mortality rate (7 versus 100% of mortality for unoperated patients) [8].

Finally, surgery remains superior to optimal medical management even though the patient is unstable, in coma or over 80.

2.2 Long-term mortality statistics and causes

Even if the TAAD is an acute disease necessitating emergency treatment, this pathology presents an important long-term morbi-mortality. Thus, 10 years survival is between 50 and 70% [3, 9, 10], and 10 years re-operation rate is around 15% [11].

Several factors contribute to this excess morbi-mortality. In Tanaka's study [12], 243 patients were operated on for TAAD, and mortality causes at follow up were cancer, heart disease and acute aortic rupture for, respectively, 37, 23 and 13% of the cases. The reoperation rate for aortic aneurysm was 5.7%. These results are similar to Kirsch's outcomes in his 2002 study [11].

Even if cancer and heart diseases cannot be decreased by the initial surgical strategy, death by acute aortic rupture and reoperation for aortic aneurysm could be prevented by the first surgery. Within this framework, the question is raised to treat not only the immediate complications of the aortic dissection but also to perform an optimal aortic repair in order to prevent long-term complications of the TAAD.

3. Ensure a durable repair

The main objective of the surgical treatment is to ensure the patient's survival. Thus, the replacement of the ascending aorta containing the primary tear and the re-establishment of the dominant flow through the true lumen prevent from acute aortic rupture and mostly correct vascular complications [13].

As seen before, the secondary objective of the surgical treatment is now to provide the best repair in order to prevent complications on the aortic valve and on the aorta. The challenge is to complete this preventing treatment without compromising the short-term survival. In this context, the European Society of Cardiology (ESC) provided recommendations upon the surgical treatment of the TAAD.

3.1 Proximal segment of the ascending aorta

- Concerning the aortic root management, the discussion is to identify the patients who need an aortic root replacement and the patients who need a more conservative aortic root treatment.

- As reported by the analysis of the International Registry of Acute Dissection (IRAD), aortic root replacement compared with conservative root management is not associated with increased inhospital mortality. Thus, the comparison based on 1995 patients found 18% of hospital mortality in root replacement group and 21.3% of hospital mortality in conservative root group (odds ratio [OR], 0.989; 95% CI, 0.710–1.379; $P = 0.949$ after covariate adjustment) [14]. Midterms observations at 3 years did not showed statistical difference between the two techniques concerning overall mortality (91.6 ± 1.3% survival for conservative root management, 92.5 ± 1.7% survival for aortic root replacement management, $P = 0.623$) and freedom from reintervention (99.3 ± 0.1% for conservative root group and 99.2 ± 0.1% for root replacement group $P = 0.770$). However, aortic root replacement must not be performed systematically. Thus, the latter is recommended for patients with sinuses of Valsalva involved by the dissection and for patients who need surgery on the aortic valve. An aortic root replacement is also recommended for patients with aneurysmal evolution risk factors such as Marfan's syndrome, increased sinuses of Valsalva diameter, and young patients.

Several techniques are suitable for aortic root replacement. In this situation, the aortic valve is the key factor.

- In most cases, the valve is normal, and a simple regurgitation by annulus enlargement is observed. Then, an aortic valve sparing repair is recommended [15]. As shown by Farhat [16], aortic valve sparing repair procedure did not show higher short-term and mid-term mortality rate compared with conservative management and Bentall procedure (15.7% for inhospital mortality and 84.7% survival at 1 year after David procedure). If initially two techniques were applied, the remodeling technique as described by Yacoub and the reimplantation technique described by David, the latter seems superior, mainly concerning the low reoperation rate [17] (**Figure 1**). Indeed, Leyh on a series of 30 patients found a 95 ± 5% freedom from reoperation in reimplantation group (David procedure) versus a 38 ± 23% remodeling group (Yacoub procedure) (P = 0.13). Yet, the cutoff for reintervention for secondary aortic insufficiency in the remodeling group was an annulus diameter over 27 mm at the time of the surgery, regardless to an associated aortic insufficiency.

- When the valve is pathological or in case of bicuspid aortic valve, an aortic valve replacement using a Bentall technique is recommended (**Figure 2**).

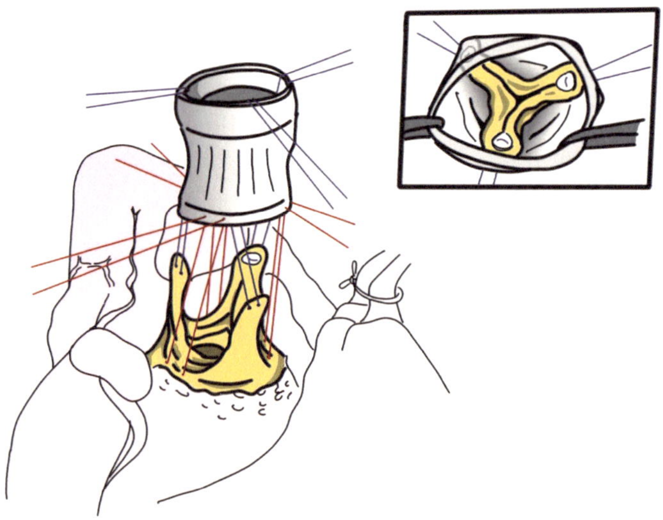

Figure 1.
David procedure.

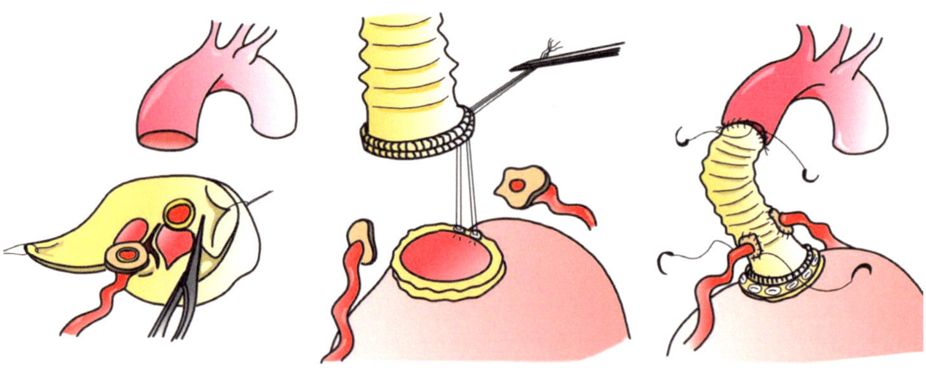

Figure 2.
Bentall procedure.

- Without aortic valve regurgitation, when the dissection does not involve the sinus of Valsalva, a simple aortic replacement with a composite graft tube can be performed.

Reimplantation valve sparing aortic root replacement (David procedure) consists of replacing the aortic root by composite graft without replacing the aortic valve. The coronary ostia are also reimplanted into the graft. This technique treats aortic regurgitation caused by annulus enlargement.

Bentall procedure involves aortic valve replacement using an aortic valve prosthesis and an aortic root replacement using a composite graft. The coronary ostia are reimplanted into the graft.

3.2 Distal segment of the ascending aorta

Whatever the extension of the repair, the distal anastomosis has to be performed without aortic clamping, under circulatory arrest [15] (ESC 2014 class 1 recommendation). Neurological protection can be provided either by deep or moderate hypothermia. If deep hypothermia (under 22°C) has been performed for decades, recently, several studies such as El-Sayed have demonstrated that moderate hypothermia at 28°C associated with anterograde cerebral perfusion was able to ensure good neurological and visceral protection. This technique provides a low rate of postoperative neurological complications (6%) within a limited cardiopulmonary bypass time (183 +/− 56 minutes) [18].

In its guidelines, the European Society of Cardiology does not recommend a type of hypothermia [15]. Nevertheless, good results of moderate hypothermia in combination with anterograde cerebral perfusion should enable generalization of this approach.

The main question for this repair is to determine how far the repair has to be performed.

Several factors will have an influence on the length of the reparation:

- The localization of the primary tear
    - The localization of the primary tear is performed by computed tomography (CT) or magnetic resonance imaging (MRI) but should be confirmed by peroperative findings. Thus, a cross clamped aorta does not allow the inspection of the aortic arch. For this reason, an open distal anastomosis is mandatory.
    - The primary tear is localized in the aortic arch in 30% of the cases of TAAD [19]. In this case, the discussion is to identify patients who need a hemiarch replacement and those who need a complete aortic arch replacement, with or without a frozen elephant trunk. The analysis of the German Registry for Acute Aortic Dissection Type A (GERAADA) demonstrated that complete aortic arch replacement compared with hemiarch replacement neither increases the in-hospital mortality (25.7 vs. 18.7% $P = 0.067$) nor the onset of new neurological deficit (12.5 vs. 13.6% $P = 0.78$) [20]. Concerning the long-term follow-up, Di Eusenio did not show any statistical difference between total arch replacement and conservative arch management [21]. Thus, 7-year survival hazard ratio was equal to 1.001 ($P = 0.8$), and freedom from aortic reintervention was equal to 1.507 ($P = 0.4$). These results are similar to other studies on the subject [22]. As a conclusion, there is no difference concerning the short- and

long-term mortality or freedom from aortic reintervention. Thus, when the entry tear is localized in the aortic arch, a total aortic arch replacement could be reasonably performed.

- In some cases, the primary tear is localized in the descending thoracic aorta, and the ascending aorta is affected by a retrograde dissection. A hybrid surgery using a frozen elephant trunk technique is the best way to manage this situation. A two-time procedure can also be performed by the realization of a complete arch repair followed by the implantation of an endoprosthesis in the descending thoracic aorta through a femoral approach.

• The presence of a malperfusion syndrome

- Malperfusion syndrome has two origins: dynamic malperfusion secondary to compression of the true lumen by the false lumen and static malperfusion secondary to the extension of the dissection into the branch vessel. In many cases of malperfusion syndromes, these two mechanisms are combined (**Figure 3a**).

Concerning the management of the malperfusion syndrome, two strategies can be applied: performing digestive endovascular (fenestration or branch stenting) reperfusion before the ascending aorta repair or conversely performing ascending aorta repair first and treat only persistent malperfusion syndrome.

Regarding the first strategy, Yamashiro [23] showed upon a short series of 10 patients with visceral malperfusion, the advantages of performing visceral arterial branch bypass before central repair, and cardiopulmonary bypass. Others suggest performing a fenestration of the intimal flap rather than abdominal open surgery. Thus, Kamman [24] provide a patient-specific algorithm suggesting treating malperfusion syndrome first, waiting for the resolution of the malperfusion, and then performing central repair. This algorithm is based upon several studies which show the poor survival rate of TAAD complicated with malperfusion syndrome especially for patients with mesenteric ischemia requiring surgery (63.2 versus 23.8% $P < 0.001$) [25]. Nevertheless, this delaying strategy is questionable since it is associated with a high mortality rate. Thus, a large proportion of patients (33% in Patel series [26], 40% in Yang series [27]) die from aortic rupture or organ failure before the central repair.

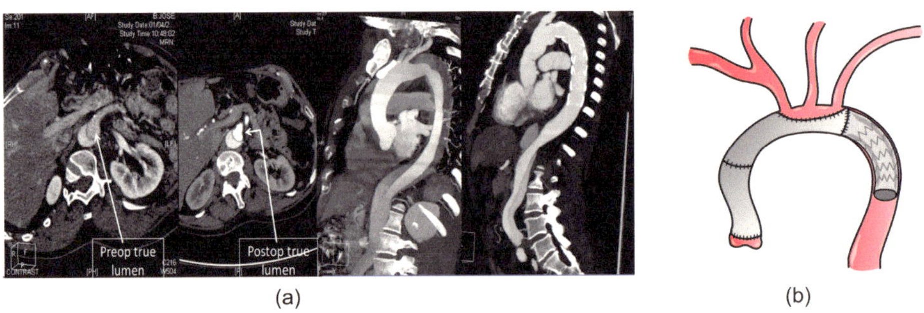

Figure 3.
(a) Type A aortic dissection complicated by malperfusion syndrome. (A) Preoperative CT: type A aortic dissection: low opacification of the true lumen with an impaired vascularization of the superior mesenteric artery. (B) Postoperative CT: type A aortic dissection treated by frozen elephant trunk: improvement of the mesenteric artery CT signal. (b) Frozen elephant trunk procedure: (A) frozen elephant trunk implantation scheme. E-vita open prothesis.

Concerning the second strategy, many authors [28, 29] propose to close the primary tear first. This approach, by redirecting the flow into the true lumen, decreases the need for latter revascularization, since in many cases the malperfusion syndrome is mainly dynamic. In Geirsson series [4], only 62.5% of patients with coronary malperfusion required coronary artery bypass and 42.9% of patients, with limb ischemia required distal revascularization after central repair. These results were similar in Charlton's study [5].

Regard to the central repair, a hybrid approach using the frozen elephant trunk technique or a two-time surgery extends the true lumen, decreases the false lumen diameter, the global aortic diameter, and creates a thrombosis of the false lumen [30] (**Figure 3b**). Thus, the vascular group of the European Association for Cardiac-Thoracic Surgery (EACTS) provided a IIa class recommendation for the use of frozen elephant trunk technique in TAAD with primary tear localized in the distal aortic arch or in the proximal half of the descending thoracic aorta in order to treat or prevent a malperfusion syndrome [31].

- The prevention of aneurysm formation

As seen before, aneurysm formation is one of the main causes of excess mortality and reoperation in patients with history of TAAD [12]. Thus, preventing this complication is an important objective of the TAAD management. To answer this issue, two surgical techniques using hybrid surgery exist:

- The frozen elephant trunk technique. This surgery includes a total arch replacement associated to a per-procedural stent delivery through the aortic true lumen. Concerning the prevention of aneurysm formation in the descending thoracic aorta, Uchida [32] proved the superiority of this technique compared with ascending aortic replacement or hemiarch replacement. Thus, he observed a decrease of late thoracic aorta event (95.7 *vs* 73.0% $P = 0.01$) mainly induced by thrombosis of the false lumen (100% of thrombosis in frozen elephant trunk group *vs* 29% in the other group). However, some limits persist concerning the frozen elephant trunk technique: this surgery is demanding, emphasize the operative time, and require experimented surgeon. Moreover, some series have shown an increasing of neurological complications [33].

- A two-time surgery including a complete aortic arch replacement followed by the implantation of an endoprothesis in the descending thoracic aorta through a femoral artery. A matter of debate is the moment of the second intervention. Most teams perform MRI or CT control till reaching aortic diameter superior to 55 mm. This approach can be discussed. Indeed, as demonstrated by the *Society of Thoracic Surgeons Endovascular Surgery Task Force,* intimal flap fibrosis appears over time [21]. This fibrosis jeopardizes endovascular treatment and frequently leads to open surgery [34]. Moreover, actual guidelines for aortic aneurysm treatment are the same whatever the etiology: at the descending thoracic aorta: a maximal diameter superior to 60 mm for open surgery and 55 mm for endovascular treatment [35]. Unfortunately, this cutoff is not suitable to dissected aorta which is a fragilized vessel. For example, Kimura found a median diameter before aortic rupture at 56 mm [36] in patient with history of TAAD.

Yet, performing a hybrid surgery in the descending thoracic aorta does not prevent in all cases from aneurysm formation. At the thoracic level, false lumen

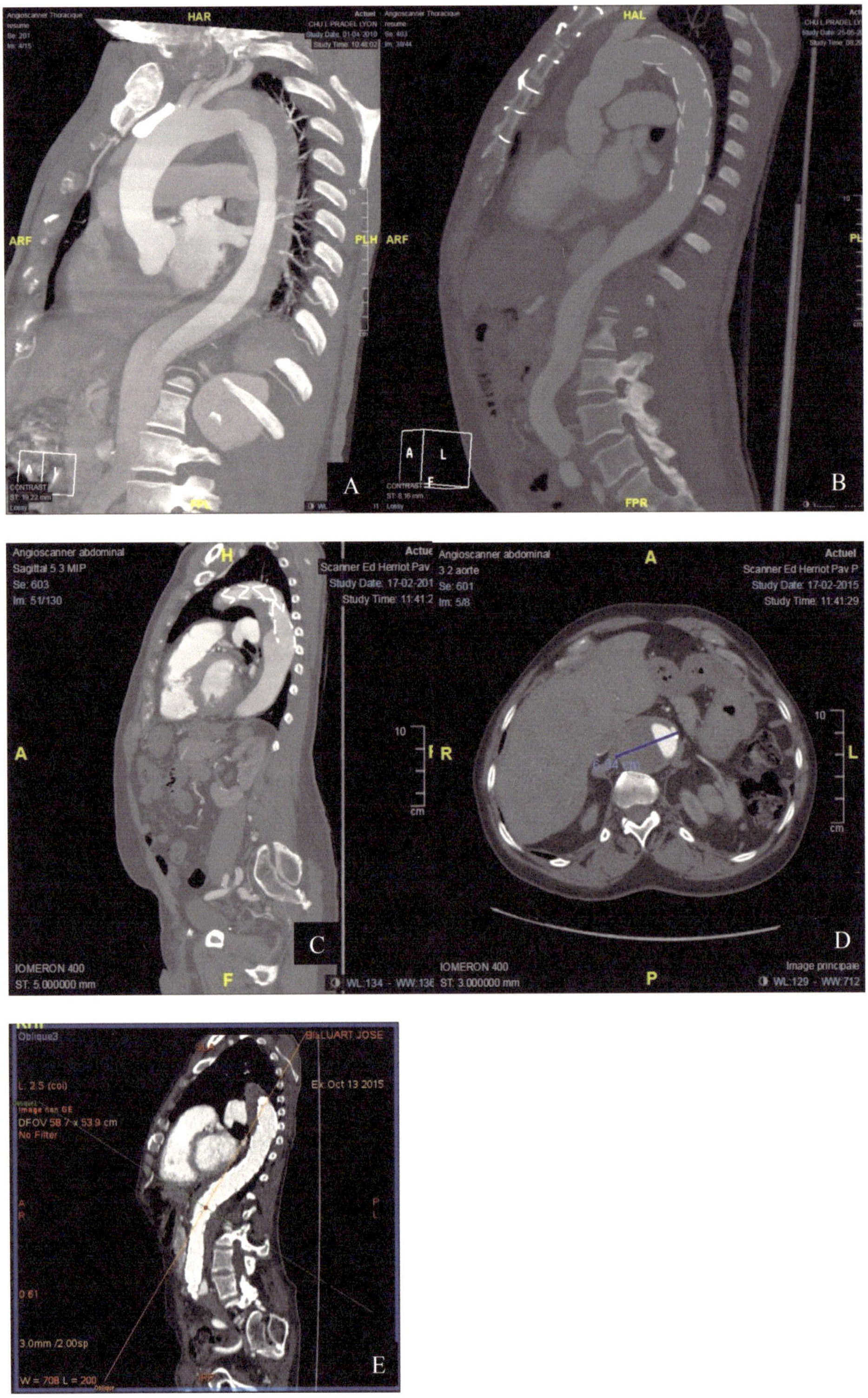

Figure 4.

Aneurysmal evolution after frozen elephant trunk procedure. (A) Preoperative CT of a type A aortic dissection. (B) Postoperative CT after frozen elephant trunk implantation (E-vita open prothesis). (C and D) 5 years postoperative. CT: Aneurysmal evolution on the descending aorta at the thoraco abdominal junction despite the thrombosis of the false lumen at the thoracic stage. (E) CT post fenestrated aortic stent graft implantation.

thrombosis induces inflammatory reaction inside the aortic wall. This inflammation is problematic; indeed, several studies have demonstrated the role of this inflammatory state in aneurysm progression, particularly through the production of metalloproteases and proinflammatory cytokines [37], these two elements leading to neo-angiogenesis and destruction of the extracellular matrix in the aortic wall. At the abdominal level, aortic aneurysm is frequently observed after hybrid surgery of dissected thoracic aorta (**Figure 4**). Several factors explain this evolution: a patent false lumen at this level, the modification of the aortic wall shear stress, the creation of a helicoidal flow downstream the endoprosthesis [38] (**Figure 5**).

To prevent this complication, Matalanis [39] proposes to perform a total aortic repair combining surgical ascending aorta repair and endovascular treatment of the descending aorta. This last treatment includes the deployment of a covered stent graft in the proximal part of descending aorta and rupture of the intimal flap for the last part of the aorta (Sabilize approach). This rupture is performed through the deployment and the dilatation under balloon of uncovered stent graft. Thus, a unique aortic channel is created, avoiding aneurysmal evolution of the false channel. Even if this technique seems appealing, reservations with regards persist. Indeed, according to Matalanis study, this technique provides specific complications such as additional visceral stenting (40% of cases), iliac stenting (20% of cases), and reintervention for endoleak (20% of cases). Moreover, only 53% had a complete false lumen thrombosis. Finally, as yet there is no long-term follow-up concerning the aortic dimension (median follow-up: 26 month) [40].

As we see, if surgical solutions exist, the prevention of aneurysm formation in the descending thoracic aorta using hybrid surgery is still discussed. Thus, the European Association for Cardio-Thoracic surgery expresses only a class IIb recommendation with a C level of evidence for this indication.

In this context, this surgery must be provided to selected patients. In order to identify which patients should be considered for a frozen elephant trunk implantation, several studies have searched for risk factor of aneurysm formation after TAAD [41, 42]. In 2003, Yeh from a series of 144 patients operated for TAAD

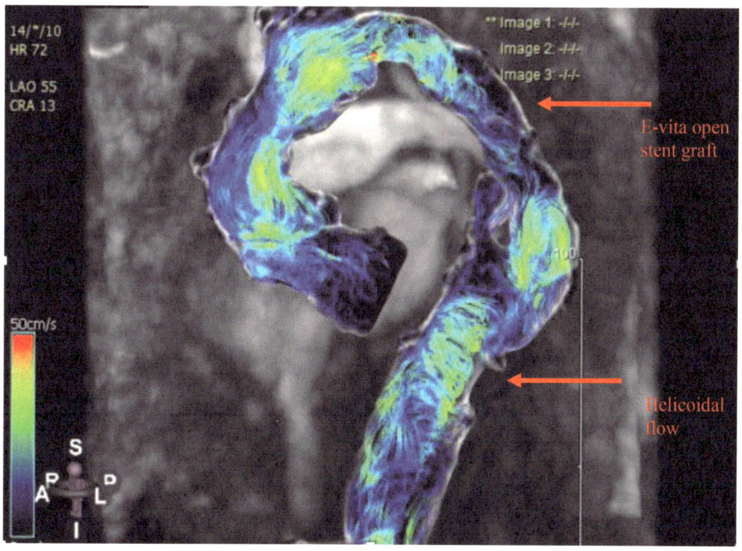

Figure 5.
4D phase-contrast MRI after treatment of a type A aortic dissection by frozen elephant trunk.

with a 3 years follow-up showed that preoperative isthmic diameter enlargement (OR = 1.11, $P = 0.0025$) and patent false lumen (OR = 13.28, $P = 0.002$) were risk factors for aneurysmal evolution [28]. Kirsch, with a longer follow-up, found a 56.1 ± 9.4% rate of reinterventions at 15 years. About 84.2% of these reinterventions were the consequence of aneurysmal evolution. After multivariate analysis, risk factors appeared to be youth, recent intervention, and type 1 dissection. Finally, the literature analysis identifies patent false lumen, preoperative isthmus diameter enlargement, preoperative descending thoracic aorta diameter enlargement over 40 mm, and long-term uncontrolled blood pressure as risk factors for descending thoracic aorta aneurysm.

Performing a descending thoracic aorta treatment by hybrid approach at the initial phase, in selected patient, could be a solution for reduction of excess mortality and morbidity of this population. Thus, patients presenting a TAAD with a descending thoracic aorta diameter superior to 40 mm could benefit from a hybrid treatment of this aortic segment.

Finally, in case of chronic dissection with aneurismal evolution reaching both ascending and thoracic descending aorta, two techniques can be discussed: a two-stage technique combining surgery on the ascending aorta via sternotomy and endovascular treatment of the descending aorta or a one-stage technique via bilateral thoracotomy (clamshell incision), with right subclavian and femoral perfusions and deep hypothermic circulatory arrest, allowing the replacement of the ascending, arch and descending aorta at different levels as described by Kouchoukos [43]. This last procedure provides low complications rates (mortality: 2.5%, reoperation for bleeding: 7.5%, neurological event: 2.4%) and a freedom from reoperation rate at 10 years equal to 84.4%.

It is important to remind that this preventive treatment has to be integrated in a global management, involving medical and surgical care, including genetic screening and strict blood pressure control. Eggebrecht demonstrated that a large part of patients with aortic dissection history (40%) had resistant hypertension despite multiple drug therapy [44], especially when patients were young and obese. These results underline the necessity to refer these patients to specialists in hypertension. Furthermore, the large number of loss of view in series [19] demonstrates that TAAD is still considered merely as an acute disease. This vision is mistaken: aortic dissection is a chronic disease, beginning in an acute way, reaching the entire aorta and requiring medical and surgical long-term follow-up.

Visualization of the aortic flow through the streamline technique: Presence of a helicoidal flow downstream the endoprosthesis.

- The surgeon's experience

The surgeon's experience is a key element of the surgical management. TAAD is a challenging pathology requiring complex surgical techniques such as aortic valve sparing and frozen elephant trunk implantation. If the operator is not familiar with aortic valve sparing repair, it is suitable to perform a Bentall intervention instead. In the same idea, performing an arch replacement followed by an endoprosthesis implantation in the descending aorta can be preferred to a frozen elephant trunk approach.

3.3 Type B aortic dissection with arch extension

Type B aortic dissection (TBAD) with retrograde arch extension occurs in 25% of cases of TBAD [45]. However, even if this situation is not rare, there are no recommendations concerning the management of this case.

Tsai [46] analyzed the International Registry of Acute Dissection Database. He found that patients with TBAD and arch extension received the same treatment than pure TBAD: medical treatment when there was no complication and endovascular or surgical treatment in case of complication. Open surgery on the aortic arch was performed in case of complication related with arch pathology: aortic arch expansion, aortic arch rupture, or malperfusion in the arch vessels. In comparison with TBAD without arch extension, mortality rates between the two groups were similar (short-term: $P = 0.61$, long-term: $P = 0.82$).

When surgery on the aortic arch is necessary, total arch replacement with frozen elephant trunk seems to be the best option. Indeed, this technique enables the aortic arch to be replaced and the primary tear to be closed when it is situated in the proximal part of the thoracic descending aorta. Moreover, an endoprothesis can be deployed in a second time if the primary tear is not occluded by the frozen elephant trunk.

Finally, TBAD with arch extension should be treated as TBAD. Aortic arch replacement combined with frozen elephant trunk should be performed in case of complication related with an arch pathology.

4. Conclusion

TAAD is a serious condition requiring emergency surgical treatment. If saving the patient remains the main objective of the surgery, long-term follow-up leads us to improve initial surgical treatment, mainly to prevent long-term aneurysmal evolution, either on the aortic root or on the descending thoracic aorta. Concerning the proximal segment, guidelines are clear: aortic root has to be replaced if the sinuses of Valsalva are involved by the dissection. Concerning the descending thoracic aorta, there is still no consensus, but studies show that hybrid surgery should be performed in case of malperfusion syndrome and when patients presents high risk factors for aneurysmal evolution.

Author details

Benoit Cosset, Sarah Abdellaoui, Hugo Huvelle, Amine Fikani and Fadi Farhat*
Department of Cardiovascular Surgery B, Hospital Louis Pradel, Hospices Civils de Lyon, Université Lyon 1, Lyon, France

*Address all correspondence to: fadi.farhat@chu-lyon.fr

References

[1] Trimarchi S, Eagle KA, Nienaber CA, Rampoldi V, Jonker FHW, De Vincentiis C, et al. Role of age in acute type A aortic dissection outcome: Report from the international registry of acute aortic dissection (IRAD). The Journal of Thoracic and Cardiovascular Surgery. 2010;**140**:784-789

[2] Berretta P, Patel H, Gleason T, Sundt M, Myrmel T, Desai N, et al. IRAD experience on surgical type A acute dissection patients: Results and predictors of mortality. Annals of Cardiothoracic Surgery. 2016;**5**:346-351

[3] Chiappini B, Schepens M, Tan E, Dell'Amore A, Morshuis W, Dossche K, et al. Early and late outcomes of acute type A aortic dissection: Analysis of risk factors in 487 consecutive patients. European Heart Journal. 2005;**26**:180-186

[4] Jex RK, Schaff HV, Piehler JM, Orszulak TA, Puga FJ, King RM, et al. Repair of ascending aortic dissection. Influence of associated aortic valve insufficiency on early and late results. The Journal of Thoracic and Cardiovascular Surgery. 1987;**93**:375-384

[5] Erbel R, Oelert H, Meyer J, Puth M, Mohr-Katoly S, Hausmann D, et al. Effect of medical and surgical therapy on aortic dissection evaluated by transesophageal echocardiography. Implications for prognosis and therapy. The European Cooperative Study Group on Echocardiography. Circulation. 1993;**87**:1604-1615

[6] Tsukube T, Hayashi T, Kawahira T, Haraguchi T, Matsukawa R, Kozawa S, et al. Neurological outcomes after immediate aortic repair for acute type A aortic dissection complicated by coma. Circulation. 2011;**124** (11 Suppl):S163-S167

[7] Pocar M, Passolunghi D, Moneta A, Mattioli R, Donatelli F. Coma might not preclude emergency operation in acute aortic dissection. The Annals of Thoracic Surgery. 2006;**81**(4):1348-1351

[8] Estrera AL, Garami Z, Miller CC, Porat EE, Achouh PE, Dhareshwar J, et al. Acute type A aortic dissection complicated by stroke: Can immediate repair be performed safely? The Journal of Thoracic and Cardiovascular Surgery. 2006;**132**(6):1404-1408

[9] Sabik JF, Lytle BW, Blackstone EH, McCarthy PM, Loop FD, Cosgrove DM. Long-term effectiveness of operations for ascending aortic dissections. The Journal of Thoracic and Cardiovascular Surgery. 2000;**119**:946-962

[10] Castrovinci S, Pacini D, Di Marco L, Berretta P, Cefarelli M, Murana G, et al. Surgical management of aortic root in type A acute aortic dissection: A propensity-score analysis. European Journal of Cardio-Thoracic Surgery. 2016;**50**:223-229

[11] Kirsch M, Soustelle C, Houel R, Hillion ML, Loisance D. Risk factor analysis for proximal and distal reoperations after surgery for acute type A aortic dissection. The Journal of Thoracic and Cardiovascular Surgery. 2002;**123**:318-325

[12] Tanaka M, Kimura N, Yamaguchi A, Adachi H. In-hospital and long-term results of surgery for acute type A aortic dissection: 243 consecutive patients. Annals of Thoracic and Cardiovascular Surgery. 2012;**18**:18-23

[13] Westaby S, Saito S, Katsumata T. Acute type A dissection: Conservative methods provide consistently low mortality. The Annals of Thoracic Surgery. 2002;**73**:707-713

[14] Di Eusanio M, Trimarchi S, Peterson MD, et al. Root replacement surgery versus more conservative management during type A acute aortic dissection repair. The Annals of Thoracic Surgery. 2014;**98**:2078-2084

[15] Erbel R, Aboyans V, Boileau C, Bossone E, Di Bartolomeo R, Aggebrecht H, et al. 2014 guidelines on the diagnosis and treatment of aortic diseases. European Heart Journal. 2014;**35**:2873-2926

[16] Farhat F, Bejan-Angoulvant T, Abdallah H, Jegaden O. Reimplantation valve sparing procedure in type A aortic dissection: A predictive factor of mortality and morbidity? In: Grundmann R, editor. Diagnosis and Treatment of Abdominal and Thoracic Aortic Aneurysms Including the Ascending Aorta and the Aortic Arch. Rijeka, Croatia: IntechOpen; 2011

[17] Leyh RG, Fischer S, Kallenbach K, Kofidis T, Pethig K, Harringer W, et al. High failure rate after valve-sparing aortic root replacement using the "remodeling technique" in acute type A aortic dissection. Circulation. 2002;**106**(12 Suppl 1):I229-I233

[18] El-Sayed Ahmad A, Papadopoulos N, Risteski P, Moritz A, Zierer A. The standardized concept of moderate-to-mild (≥28°C) systemic hypothermia during selective antegrade cerebral perfusion for all-comers in aortic arch surgery: Single-center experience in 587 consecutive patients over a 15-year period. The Annals of Thoracic Surgery. 2017;**104**(1):49-55

[19] Bachet J, Goudot B, Dreyfus G. Surgery for acute type A aortic dissection: The Hopital Foch experience (1977-1998). The Annals of Thoracic Surgery. 1999;**67**:2006-2009

[20] Easo J, Weigang E, Hölzl PPF, Horst M, Hoffmann I, Blettner M, et al. Influence of operative strategy for the aortic arch in DeBakey type I aortic dissection: Analysis of the German registry for acute aortic dissection type a. The Journal of Thoracic and Cardiovascular Surgery. 2012;**144**:617-623

[21] Svensson LG, Kouchoukos NT, Miller DC, Bavaria JE, Coselli JS, Curi MA, et al. Expert consensus document on the treatment of descending thoracic aortic disease using endovascular stent-grafts. Society of Thoracic Surgeons endovascular surgery task force. The Annals of Thoracic Surgery 2008;**85**(1 Suppl):S1-41

[22] Di Eusanio M, Berretta P, Cefarelli M, Jacopo A, Murana G, Castrovinci S, et al. Total arch replacement versus more conservative management in type A acute aortic dissection. The Annals of Thoracic Surgery. 2015;**100**(1):88-94

[23] Li B, Ma W-G, Liu Y-M, Sun L-Z. Is extended arch replacement justified for acute type A aortic dissection? Interactive Cardiovascular and Thoracic Surgery. 2015;**20**(1):120-126

[24] Yamashiro S, Arakaki R, Kise Y, Inafuku H, Kuniyoshi Y. Management of visceral malperfusion complicated with acute type A aortic dissection. Interactive Cardiovascular and Thoracic Surgery. 2015;**21**(3):346-351

[25] Kamman AV, Yang B, Kim KM, Williams DM, Michael Deeb G, Patel HJ. Visceral malperfusion in aortic dissection: The michigan experience. Seminars in Thoracic and Cardiovascular Surgery. 2017;**29**(2):173-178

[26] Di Eusanio M, Trimarchi S, Patel HJ, Hutchison S, Suzuki T, Peterson MD, et al. Clinical presentation, management, and short-term outcome of patients with type A acute dissection complicated by mesenteric malperfusion: Observations from

the international registry of acute aortic dissection. The Journal of Thoracic and Cardiovascular Surgery. 2013;**145**(2):385-390.e1

[27] Patel HJ, Williams DM, Dasika NL, Suzuki Y, Deeb GM. Operative delay for peripheral malperfusion syndrome in acute type A aortic dissection: A long-term analysis. The Journal of Thoracic and Cardiovascular Surgery. 2008;**135**(6):1288-1295-1296

[28] Geirsson A, Szeto WY, Pochettino A, McGarvey ML, Keane MG, Woo YJ, et al. Significance of malperfusion syndromes prior to contemporary surgical repair for acute type A dissection: Outcomes and need for additional revascularizations. European Journal of Cardio-Thoracic Surgery. 2007;**32**(2):255-262

[29] Charlton-Ouw KM, Sandhu HK, Leake SS, Jeffress K, Miller CC, Durham CA, et al. Need for limb revascularization in patients with acute aortic dissection is associated with mesenteric ischemia. Annals of Vascular Surgery. 2016;**36**:112-120

[30] Takagi H, Umemoto T, the ALICE Group. A meta-analysis of total arch replacement with frozen elephant trunk in acute type A aortic dissection. Vascular and Endovascular Surgery. 2016;**50**:33-46

[31] Shrestha M, Bachet J, Bavaria J, Carrel TP, De Paulis R, Di Bartolomeo R, et al. Current status and recommendations for use of the frozen elephant trunk technique: A position paper by the vascular domain of EACTS. European Journal of Cardio-Thoracic Surgery. 2015;**47**:759-769

[32] Uchida N, Shibamura H, Katayama A, Shimada N, Sutoh M, Ishihara H. Operative strategy for acute type A aortic dissection: Ascending aortic or hemiarch versus total arch replacement with frozen elephant trunk. The Annals of Thoracic Surgery. 2009;**87**:773-777

[33] Yan Y, Xu L, Zhang H, Xu ZY, Ding XY, Wang SW, et al. Proximal aortic repair versus extensive aortic repair in the treatment of acute type A aortic dissection: A meta-analysis. European Journal of Cardio-Thoracic Surgery. 2016;**49**:1392-1401

[34] Abraha I, Romagnoli C, Montedori A, Cirocchi R. Thoracic stent graft versus surgery for thoracic aneurysm. Cochrane Database of Systematic Reviews. 2016;**6**:CD006796

[35] Svensson LG, Kouchoukos NT, Miller DC, Bavaria JE, Coselli JS, Curi MA, et al. Expert consensus document on the treatment of descending thoracic aortic disease using endovascular stent-grafts. The Annals of Thoracic Surgery. 2008;**85**:S1-S41

[36] Kimura N, Itoh S, Yuri K, Adachi K, Matsumoto H, Yamaguchi A, et al. Reoperation for enlargement of the distal aorta after initial surgery for acute type A aortic dissection. The Journal of Thoracic and Cardiovascular Surgery. 2015;**149**(2 Suppl):S91-S98

[37] Cifani N, Proietta M, Tritapepe L, Di Gioia C, Ferri L, Taurino M, et al. Stanford-a acute aortic dissection, inflammation, and metalloproteinases: A review. Annals of Medicine. 2015;**47**:441-446

[38] Clough RE, Waltham M, Giese D, Taylor PR, Schaeffer T. A new imaging method for assessment of aortic dissection using four-dimensional phase contrast magnetic resonance imaging. Journal of Vascular Surgery. 2012;**55**:914-923

[39] Matalanis G, Ip S. A new paradigm in the management of acute type A aortic dissection: Total aortic repair. The Journal of Thoracic and Cardiovascular Surgery. 2019;**157**(1):3-11

[40] Girardi LN. Is a more extensive operation justified for acute type A dissection repair? The Journal of Thoracic and Cardiovascular Surgery. 2019;**157**(1):12-13

[41] Almeida AG, Nobre AL, Pereira RA, Costa-Pereira A, Tavares C, Cravino J, et al. Impact of aortic dimensions and pulse pressure on late aneurysm formation in operated type A aortic dissection. A magnetic resonance imaging study. The International Journal of Cardiovascular Imaging. 2008;**24**:633-640

[42] Yeh C-H, Chen M-C, Wu Y-C, Wang Y-C, Chu J-J, Lin PJ. Risk factors for descending aortic aneurysm formation in medium-term follow-up of patients with type A aortic dissection. Chest. 2003;**124**:989-995

[43] Kouchoukos NT, Kulik A, Castner CF. Clinical outcomes and rates of aortic growth and reoperation after 1-stage repair of extensive chronic thoracic aortic dissection. The Journal of Thoracic and Cardiovascular Surgery. 2018;**155**(5):1926-1935

[44] Eggebrecht H, Schmermund A, von Birgelen C, Naber CK, Bartel T, Wenzel RR, Erbel R. Resistant hypertension in patients with chronic aortic dissection. Journal of Human Hypertension 2005;19:227-231

[45] Estrera AL, Miller CC, Safi HJ, Goodrick JS, Keyhani A, Porat EE, et al. Outcomes of medical management of acute type B aortic dissection. Circulation. 2006;**114**(1 Suppl):I384-I389

[46] Tsai TT, Isselbacher EM, Trimarchi S, Bossone E, Pape L, Januzzi JL, et al. Acute type B aortic dissection: Does aortic arch involvement affect management and outcomes? Insights from the international registry of acute aortic dissection (IRAD). Circulation. 2007;**116**(11 Suppl): I150-I156